IMPOTENCY is a problem affecting millions of men in America, maybe as many as 20 million. About 90% of these men are unable to achieve erections because of physical reasons. Others, because of mental reasons.

Almost all men, at one time or another, have had an incident of erectile failure. Occasional impotence can be provoked by a variety of causes such as anxiety, alcohol or fatigue. This temporary impotence will pass and does not require therapy.

If the impotence persists over three months it can be considered chronic, and medical help is available. Chronic impotence is the inability to achieve and maintain an erection over a prolonged period of time.

Although we're both medical doctors, we made this book easy to read for the non-medical professional. It's written by doctors but not (especially) for doctors. It is meant to explain to you what your problem might be and how it can be remedied.

Just know this! There is an answer and there are cures for impotency. It is not a disgrace to be in this condition; it's dumb not to do anything about it! Impotency just happens.

We wrote this book with one purpose in mind; to put both you and your partner at ease and to help you enjoy life. Impotency is (almost always) reversible!

REVERSING IMPOTENCE

FOREVER!

by

David F. Mobley, M.D., F.A.C.S.
Steven K. Wilson, M.D., F.A.C.S.

SWAN PUBLISHING
Texas • California • New York

Author(s): Dr. David F. Mobley *and* Dr. Steven K. Wilson
Editors: John Pepe *and* Pete Billac
Cover Design: Mark Fornataro
Layout Design: Sharon Davis
The Male Sexual Well-Being Series by:
Polaris Entertainment Group

REVERSING IMPOTENCE FOREVER - The Male Sexual Well-Being Series is
available in quantity discounts through SWAN Publishing Company, 126 Live
Oak, Suite 100, Alvin, TX 77511 (713)388-2547 or FAX (713)585-3738.

Printed in the United States of America

The ideas, procedures, and suggestions in this book are not intended as a
substitute for the medical advice of a trained health professional. All matters
regarding our health require medical supervision. Consult your physician before
adopting the suggestions in the book, as well as any condition that may require
diagnosis or medical attention. The authors and publisher disclaim any liability
arising directly or indirectly from the use of techniques in this book.

This book is dedicated to
the memory of the late

F. Brantley Scott, M.D.

Our friend and mentor and a brilliant
physician whose skills, courage and caring
has impacted the lives of hundreds of
thousands of men, women, and
children around the world.

PROLOGUE

As medical doctors, we have handled over 10,000 cases of impotence. We hear stories from people that are almost totally unbelievable, but we work towards curing them.

This book on correcting impotence is the latest as of the copyright date and some of the treatments, though seemingly somewhat complicated, are sometimes necessary. It's the best there is.

You'll notice the words "however" or "unfortunately" many times because there is no *magic pill* that can be taken to correct Impotency. We wish there were. (We will talk about one special pill that might help).

What this book will do is to enlighten you on several things. First and foremost, impotence is (almost always) reversible! The methods are the latest and the technology sound. We point out the *good* and the *bad* parts of each and then let you decide.

The most painful part of our work is the fact that so very many men put off coming to us or to other medical professionals who specialize in impotence. I bold the word "specialize" because of the thousands of urologists in the United States, a very small percentage specialize in impotence.

I'm certain there are many jokes about our profession (as there are for proctologist's and lawyers) but we're proud of what we do and we feel fulfillment in being able to change an unhappy life (sexual and otherwise) into a happy one.

From some of the case studies we list in the back of this book, you'll be able to get an idea of how tragic impotence can be—if it isn't corrected! We're hoping that this book will help you decide to take a step forward and seek medical attention that will certainly enhance your sexual capabilities and put more *pizazz* in your sex life.

I also want to explain a bit about the humor we have injected into this book. We, by no means, think any of this is funny but we also feel that a positive attitude and a sense of humor is necessary to a complete, fun-filled life. Perhaps some of this doesn't seem very funny to you now, but, once you have your problem corrected, it will!

TABLE OF CONTENTS

Chapter 1

What is Impotence?

"It's all in your head." That is what most men who suffered from impotence used to be told by their doctors. By labeling it a psychological disorder, many men with medical problems were made to feel inferior or "unmanly." The stigma attached to being impotent was so pervasive that most impotent men were reluctant to admit it, even to their doctor. Those who did were often hustled off to a psychiatrist. Impotent men were done a disservice.

Fortunately, we now know that this is seldom the case. While it *can* be a symptom of a psychological disease, new technology and diagnostic tests prove it is much more often the sign of a physical disorder. It is essential that we understand that impotence in an experienced male is seldom due to psychological reasons. In short, it's probably not "all in your head."

YOU ARE NOT ALONE

The impotent man is not alone. Impotence is a common problem. Probably more than twenty million men in the United States suffer from some form of failure to achieve or maintain an erection and the effects of impotence are often much broader and more debilitating than first believed.

Keep in mind that these numbers indicate that more than 1 in 10 men walking around are suffering from this problem. It has also been shown from a recent survey in the state of Massachusetts that somewhere in the neighborhood of 50% of men over age 40 suffer from some form of sexual dysfunction. Those of us in Texas don't believe the numbers could possibly be that high—well, not in Texas! But, woefully, they probably are.

Many men do not believe this could possibly ever happen to them, but if it does and that person is you, don't despair. It could be something easy to remedy. If not, chances are high that it can still be fixed. Stay tuned and stay positive, you're about to learn of solutions to impotence.

Men who suffer any form of impotence begin to truly worry about it. Again, it's okay because—it can be treated! Don't worry—do something about it! The ability to make love plays an important role in many men's lives as reported in the following *USA Today* survey.

We specifically requested that the following survey not include television watching to be fair to the respondent's partner. These percentages, however, show the importance making love is to many men.

Men's Favorite Home Activities

Activity	Percentage Choosing
Making love	64%
Spending time with family	56%
Listening to music	34%
Home repairs	23%
Reading	23%

Respondent could choose more than one activity.
Source: Spiegel, Inc. 1986 Survey of 476 men reported in USA Today

Because sexual intercourse is one of the basic functions in a man's life, his ability to achieve and maintain an erection can be vital to his self-esteem. The nagging thought of being unable to have or to sustain an erection cause thousands of men to avoid sexual contact. Some men will go to great lengths to cover up their impotence and many times this lack of affection is misinterpret by his partner.

Often, the afflicted man will avoid his partner, sometimes to the point of granting her a divorce or severing the relationship—anything to keep her from knowing the real truth. Impotence is not worth that kind of concern. It is usually treatable.

THE GOOD NEWS

The first step in treating impotence is that the sufferer understands this common disorder. The purpose of this book is to explain in everyday language, man's anatomy, physiology, and ability to achieve and maintain an erection. If we know how the male body functions, we can better understand the reasons for male impotence and address questions about treatment.

The good news is that all most of the causes of impotence can be treated successfully. The dark silence which has surrounded the problem of overcoming impotency has been penetrated. More and more couples are now interested in facing this disorder and are turning to professionals for help.

One of the first things we tell our patients suffering from impotence and they learn this on the very first office visit, is "you can be helped!" The chances that a man suffering from impotence cannot be helped is extremely small.

DEFINING IMPOTENCE

Before going any further, let's define impotence. *Impotency is a man's inability to gain or maintain an erection adequate for the completion of sexual intercourse.* Impotence has nothing to do with sexual desire, orgasm, ejaculation, or fertility. It is simply failure to get enough blood into the penis and hold it there with enough rigidity long enough to achieve mutually satisfying sexual intercourse.

Keep in mind that this is not an "all-or-none" phenome-non. In other words, a partial erection qualifies as impo-tence in this definition. Usually, the first step in losing erection-capability is to lose the ability to sustain the erection.

The next step is loss of the ability to get an erection at all! Somewhere along this downward, inevitable slide, most men will wonder, "What's going on here?" and the smart ones will seek medical attention.

WHO BECOMES IMPOTENT

Any male who is physically mature enough to experi-ence sexual desire can become impotent. Because the image of a desirable American male includes not only being healthy, wealthy, and attractive, but also sexually active, the pressure on a man to prove himself can be tremendous. The inability to perform sexually makes many men feel they have failed!

This can lead to feelings of inhibition, lack of self-esteem and self-condemnation. The inability to have or maintain an erection can quickly cause a constant source of unhappiness.

In the past, there has been a social stigma associated with discussing impotence with anyone, whether it be a partner, friend or doctor. Frequently, older men were told that at a certain age, normal sexual relations were no longer a part of their capabilities. This, of course, is false.

We have had men come to our office with impotence, who were told by some physicians that they were too old to expect normal function and, some of these men were in their 30's! This was absurd.

Consequently, many men who had continued sexual desires and suffered from impotence became constantly frustrated and desperate. They "went for" a variety of gimmicks and quackery! Some of the more absurd was rhinoceros horn extract, zinc, trace minerals, and a variety of so-called *love potions*.

Charlatans and fast-buck-artists have advertised in every magazine imaginable promising a cure. To the frustrated victim, any solution was welcomed. Such treatment-promises took advantage of the impotent male's desperation and had generally no medically proven success.

Keep in mind, that even though we live in a very enlightened age, these potions are still being sold. Many men turn to these cures only to incur needless expense. Some use escapist solutions such as alcohol or drugs, instead of improving the problem, which may aggravate impotence and make life even more miserable.

The only effective solution for the impotent male is to seek the advice of a medical professional! We remind men that *Love Potion Number Nine* is a song, not a pill! There is no magic pill. The closest thing we have to such a pill is *Yohimbine*, discussed later *in Chapter 5*.

Some males have *predisposing factors* that can cause premature impotence at an early age. These factors include problems with high blood pressure, hardening of the arteries (atherosclerosis), elevated cholesterol, strokes, heart problems, alcoholism, drug abuse, surgery, and disk problems in the lower back to name a few.

WHO CAN HELP

The most important step for the impotent male is to seek appropriate medical assistance from a qualified urologist who specializes in this problem. The urologist does an evaluation first, then makes tests to discover the cause of the impotence. Through physical examination and diagnostic testing, the impotence specialist can recognize symptoms, assess the cause, and treat the disorder accordingly.

Other forms of sexual dysfunction may be associated with impotence and complicate or confuse therapy. The impotence urologist is trained to distinguish *true erectile failure* from other sexual problems. All of these problems listed below, as well as failure to get an erection, can be treated by the impotence urologist.

- Painful ejaculation
- Retrograde ejaculation
- Occasional inability to achieve erection
- Sexual inability due to alcohol consumption
- Sexual inability with one partner and not another
- Premature or early ejaculation
- Lack of sexual desire
- Failure to reach orgasm

Because they are trained specifically to deal with these problems, the impotence urologist is the most cost-effective source of help. Fortunately, most insurance companies and Medicare recognize these crippling conditions and cover diagnosis and treatment.

We make somewhat of an issue here of the *impotence urologist* because it is a somewhat specialized area of urology. Many urologists are not really trained or qualified in the area of impotence. For example, in the Houston area with somewhere around 150 urologists, only a handful do a large proportion of this kind of specialty.

Whether the problem is physical or psychological, the urologist who specializes in impotence can help each man realize a more fulfilling sexual life. The sooner the patient acts, the less time he and his partner will suffer. We find that most of our patients have suffered needlessly for many years, (an average of 5 years) before seeking help. Don't you follow suit. If it bothers you and if it doesn't correct itself in a few months, get help!

If we accomplish anything at all with this book, we'd like the foremost advice to be the one you follow. Seek the help of a qualified urologist who deals with impotence—now! Immediate help is available.

Chapter 2

Male Anatomy and How It Functions

There are three separate chambers in the normal penis: two inter-connected erectile chambers called the *corpora cavernosum* which occupy the bulk of the penis, and the *urethra*, a tube which can carry either urine or semen (Fig. 1).

These erectile chambers are attached at the pubic bone and extend outward from the abdominal wall to the visible portion of the penis. This attachment helps keep the penis rigid when the chambers are filled with blood.

Each erectile chamber is made of sponge-like tissue (smooth muscle and venous lacunar space) which fills with blood during the arousal phase. The blood is trapped in the penis, expanding and hardening the penis for penetration (Fig. 2). Now that we know the structure of the penis, let's discuss its three primary functions: urination, erection, and ejaculation.

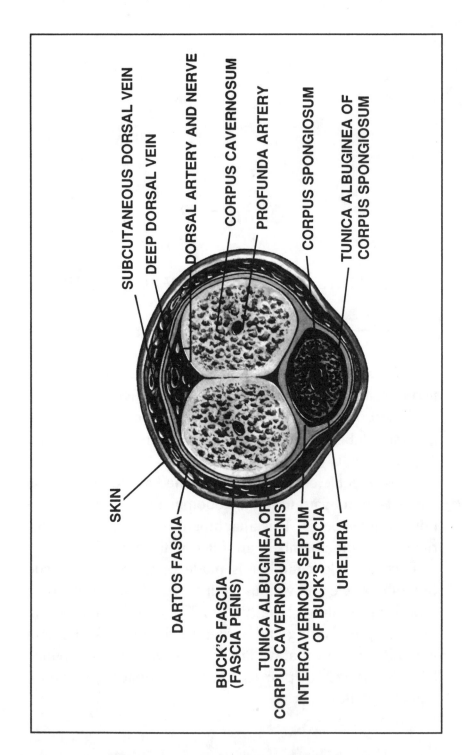

Figure 1 - "Cross Section of the Penis"

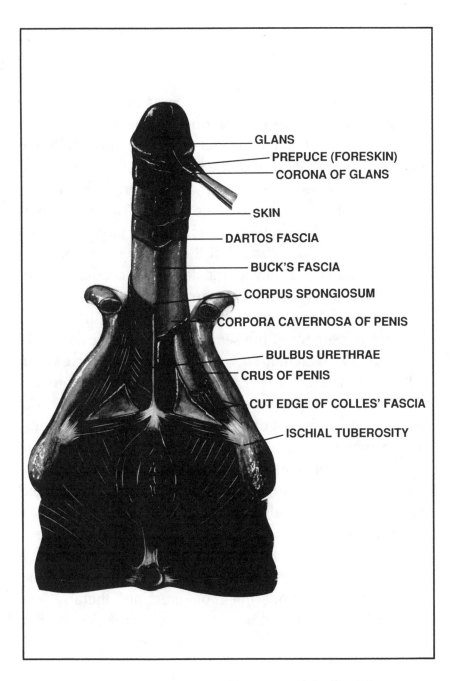

Figure 2 - "Anatomical Drawing of the Penis"

URINATION

The *urethra* is the tube in the penis that carries urine during urination, and semen during ejaculation. When the urge to urinate is felt, the bladder will empty urine into the urethra to be carried out of the body.

On its way from the bladder to the penis, the urethra must pass through the *prostate gland*. The prostate is shaped like a doughnut and the urethra passes through "the hole in the doughnut." If the prostate is enlarged it may affect a man's ability to urinate with a forcible stream.

The prostate gland plays no part in the erectile function but provides lubrication and nutrition for the sperm. Ninety-five percent of the semen is actually prostate fluid and only 3% is actual sperm. That's why a decrease in volume of the ejaculate is not noticed after vasectomy.

While the prostate has no actual function in erection of the penis, enlargement of the prostate that naturally occurs as men age, may actually inhibit erectile activity. We have noted an occasional patient whose erections improve significantly after surgical correction of their enlarged prostate. We have also found that a patient's voiding difficulty can complicate some solutions for impotence.

It is sometimes important that an enlarged prostate be treated prior to beginning some impotence therapies (e.g. surgical implants and "injection erection" therapy, see Chapter 6). A welcomed bonus is that occasionally treating the enlarged prostate may restore potency.

ERECTION

The process of erection is begun by either:

Psychogenic stimulation —thinking of a sexually
　　　arousing situation, or
Physical stimulation —touching the male anatomy
　　　in a sexual manner.

A nerve center in the brain acts on erotic thoughts while another center (in the spinal cord) responds to touching. Both work together to produce an erection as a reflex action. This reflex is assisted by the male hormone, *testosterone*, and "messenger chemicals" in the brain called *neurotransmitters*.

When one of the above two stimulations initiates an erection, the erectile chambers become engorged with blood. When a man becomes aroused, these vessels enlarge allowing blood to flow into the chambers at seven times the normal flow. As the chambers enlarge, they squeeze the small veins of the penis, trapping the blood.

Normally, the penis maintains an erection until ejaculation is completed. After orgasm, the nerve centers which started the process of erection reverse the action by constricting the blood flow into the penis. This action causes the closing pressure on the small veins to decrease, allowing the blood to flow out of the penis. When the penile compartments are devoid of extra blood, the penis is soft.

As you might suspect from reading this, you can see that the circulation of the penis is *very complicated*. When we explain this to you and are forced to use medical terminology, know that we are neither trying to impress you nor confuse you. We recognize that problems with impotency are paramount to a healthy, fun-filled life to many.

One of the circulatory systems that we hear a lot about is the circulation of the heart, but the circulation in the penis is truly much more complicated. If you stop and think about it for a second you realize that everywhere else in the body there is always a perfect balance between the blood going to an organ and the blood leaving an organ.

Your finger tips, for instance, never become firm because of more blood being "trapped" in the finger. This rapid transference occurs only in the penis and, only during an erection. Pretty amazing eh? As we often say in jest to our cardiology colleagues, *"What is the point in getting good circulation to the heart if you don't have good circulation to the penis?"*

Along the lines of this circulation issue, we should note that some men can maintain an erection after ejaculation but usually, in most men, the penis becomes flaccid (deflated) after orgasm and ejaculation.

Note that an erection must occur as a result of mental or physical stimulation. Unfortunately, it cannot be the result of sheer force of will. Many factors, both mental and physical, must function correctly to cause and maintain an erection. Nerve signals, blood vessel responses, and a fine balance of chemicals all play a part. Taking all this into consideration, plus the effect of age on the body, it is not surprising that impotency can and does occur in so many men. No wonder it is a major male concern.

Recently, *nitric oxide* was identified as the "chief

messenger" to the smooth muscle of the penis. Since nitric oxide is decreased in the penis of the impotent man, medical research is concentrating on how to utilize this chemical in the treatment of impotence. We are probably 6-10 years away from a commercial application.

EJACULATION

The sperm and prostatic fluid are channeled out of the body by the urethra during ejaculation. Produced in the testicles, sperm is transferred into the maturing center (*epididymis*) located adjacent to the testicle.

After reaching maturity, sperm travel to the base of the prostate in an organ called the *seminal vesicles,* where they remain until ejaculation. When sexual arousal and ultimately ejaculation occur, the sperm are projected through a tiny tube—the *vas deferens*—to the prostate where they are mixed with the seminal and prostatic fluids. These seminal emissions act as a lubricant and sustain the sperm during the first 36 hours of passage up the female *fallopian tube* to fertilize the egg.

During orgasm and ejaculation, the internal *sphincter* (a muscle at the base of the bladder) contracts to prevent leakage of urine. This allows for a normal flow of the ejaculate through the urethra. Following certain surgeries, an illness, or due to certain medications, this sphincter may not operate normally and remains open, and the ejaculate flows back into the bladder instead of being expelled normally. The sperm leaves the body later during urination.

This is called a *retrograde ejaculation* and it is most

commonly seen after prostate surgery, spinal cord injury, a break in the sympathetic nerve chain, or in diabetes. It may also be caused by some blood pressure medicines.

Ejaculation has nothing to do with erection! In fact, impotent men usually have no problem achieving orgasm and ejaculation with a soft penis. This means that the impotent male may experience his own sexual pleasure, but, may be is unable to provide satisfactory pleasure of intercourse for his partner.

THE INCONSISTENCY OF IMPOTENCY

Impotence is not always the same in every man. Some men will complain of failure to keep the erection, some will complain they cannot get an erection at all, and others will note they only get half an erection with failure of the penis to get hard enough to sustain penetration. Many patients will complain of all three presentations at various times in their history.

Regardless, all patients are frustrated that their erection is not predictable as it was in younger years. Keep in mind, unfortunately, we are all on a slow downhill slide called life, and facing these issues is virtually inevitable. But, it does not usually occur all at once, unless there is a severe physical trauma, fractured pelvis, or surgery. Usually it is a slow decline, with periods where things will be better and then worse, and perhaps better again for awhile.

We don't really understand this, but it is a well-recognized occurrence. However, it is important for all men— and women—to realize that the natural slide is towards increasingly poorer sexual function, until eventually it is lost altogether. But have we said this a time or two before, there is help!

PERFORMANCE ANXIETY

After a few failures at intercourse, the man may become frightened that it will fail him all the time. This fear of failure or performance anxiety, makes the physical problem worse and he begins to fail every time. The next step in this accelerating process is for the man to lose interest in sex and complain about lack of desire.

Actually, he isn't suffering from lack of desire but from lack of interest! It's a normal, everyday occurrence and we hear of it all the time from our patients. After all, who wants to play baseball if you're going to strike out every time you come to bat?

To use another sports analogy, those of you who play golf will understand. Imagine you are at the Masters. It's Sunday, the last day of the tournament and you have a putt to sink on the 18th hole and you win it all! Do you think you would be anxious? I would say so. Some men put themselves in this position sexually, and anxiety takes over—and wins!

We recommend that you try to recognize your own anxieties, and deal with them to some extent, if you can. We'll talk at greater length about professional help being available in Chapter 6.

Sexual relationships are to be enjoyed. Don't be too hard on yourself, try to enjoy the moment without too much self-pressure for the perfect performance. As one of our jocular psychology colleagues once commented, "The harder you try, the softer it gets!" Most men can relate to this.

PREMATURE EJACULATION

Some men develop premature ejaculation which means that they complete their orgasm prior to their partner's satisfaction, creating an unsatisfactory sexual relationship. One of the reasons premature ejaculation occurs is because the man rushes to orgasm out of fear that he will lose his erection.

Oftentimes, correcting the impotence thereby giving him an erection he can trust will solve this problem of early ejaculation. There are now some medications that have been shown to be somewhat successful.

Generally speaking, *retraining* is the best method. Don't rush it. Having intercourse with someone you love should be savored. If it's been a "while" since your last inter-course, premature ejaculation is understandable (and understood by your partner) but to have it happen on a regular basis is neither understood nor accepted.

"Premature ejaculation" is a very poor term. It tends to indicate that something is "wrong" with the man. There is nothing wrong that can't be corrected. What we call premature ejaculation is really *normal* ejaculation. What we want you to do is learn is to slow down ejaculation. The problem is treatable in most cases. Here's a recent example.

CASE STUDY

Ron is 45, a hard-working oil company executive, and first sought help with sexual dysfunction after having been married 18 years. The problem had been ongoing for about two years and his wife's concern led him to our office.

He said he really thought he did not have a physical problem as such. He mentioned stress of the job and family obligations were creating this "situation." He said he was losing interest in sex, and was beginning to question his masculinity. For these past two years when he and his wife had sexual relations he was having consistent premature ejaculation.

After a minimal amount of evaluation, the problem was diagnosed, and after he and his wife spent a few visits with a counselor skilled in sexual dysfunction, things were back where they should be. No medication or surgery—just talk!

Chapter 3

Physical Causes of Impotency

More than three-fourths of all impotence can be traced to a physical problem. Improper functioning of either nerves, blood vessels, hormones, or body chemicals can result in failure to achieve an erection. The most common cause of impotence is *poor penile circulation of blood.* This takes the form of failure to fill the penis with sufficient blood or failure to store the blood once the penis is filled. To simplify this, vascular impotence can be considered "failure to fill" or "failure to store."

VASCULAR INSUFFICIENCY—FAILURE TO FILL

Since it requires a seven-fold increase in the penile blood flow to achieve an erection, the blood vessels must dilate to handle the additional volume. Hardening of the arteries (arteriosclerosis) decreases the elasticity of these small arteries. The arteries are then unable to respond adequately to allow the penis to fill with blood. Diabetes, years of heavy smoking, and elevated cholesterol levels will accelerate arteriosclerosis. These conditions give the heartbreaking, but all too common, picture of vigorous men in their fifties and sixties becoming impotent.

Arteriosclerosis is a generalized disease affecting many blood vessels other than the penis. Most vascularly insufficient impotent men have some degree of hardening of the arteries all over their bodies but it is not severe enough to cause symptoms other than "failure to fill" impotence. Other impotent men have enough restriction of the heart *coronary* arteries to cause heart pain or exertion angina. Some have symptoms of impending stroke because of vascular insufficiency in the large vessels of the neck *carotid arteries.*

The same vascular insufficiency that occurs in the heart or neck also occurs in the impotent man's penile circulation. The patient with coronary insufficiency is asymptomatic at rest but develops chest pain with activity. Likewise, the patient with penile insufficiency is unable to develop erections with sexual stimulation.

Arteriosclerosis—the most common cause of impotence in men over 60 years of age

Unfortunately, hardening of the arteries is a very frequent cause of impotence. It is by far the most common cause of impotence in men over sixty. *Some investigators believe 65% of all men over 65 are impotent from vascular insufficiency.* Medical researchers know that the increase in impotence seen in older men is due to fatty cholesterol deposits in the small penile arteries. Four factors have been identified as predisposing aging men to develop poor penile circulation: high cholesterol, smoking, diabetes, and high blood pressure.

CIRCULATORY DEFICIENCIES

Young men without arteriosclerosis can also be impotent due to restrictive circulation in the penis. The deep penile arteries are only one-eighth inch in diameter. It takes very little restriction to produce a reduction in blood flow. Some men are born with inadequate penile circulation; others develop it as a result of injury.

Other times, a globule of fat may travel to the penile vessels and obstruct flow as a result of surgery or an injury distant to the penis. Microsurgical techniques can be successful in correcting this type of impotence. There are very few impotent men with these isolated lesions. The majority have generalized hardening of the arteries and are not candidates for the surgery.

VASCULAR INSUFFICIENCY—FAILURE TO STORE

THE STEAL SYNDROME

The "steal syndrome" is an arterial phenomenon which occurs during intercourse in certain positions. An erection can be achieved with sexual arousal. However, in certain sexual positions, the blood flow to the lower body and pelvic area is restricted. Blood is *stolen* from the penis, resulting in loss of erection. A simple solution is to alter positions. For example, by changing from the missionary position to his back or side, a man can avoid the constrictions placed on his hips and avoid the "steal."

ABNORMAL VENOUS DRAINAGE—VENOUS LEAKERS

Erections which are poorly maintained and which disappear quickly prior to satisfaction may be a result of abnormal venous drainage. There are several reasons for this. If the erectile chambers do not fill completely because of smooth muscle failure (nitric oxide deficiency), or leakage is caused by inadequate closing pressure on the small veins. Failure to store may also be caused by an abnormal connection between arteries and the veins of the penis directing blood away from the erectile chambers.

Finally, there may be extensive blood drainage due to extra or abnormal venous pathways. This is called *collateral circulation*. An example of this in another part of the body is varicose veins of the legs.

When the blood "leaks" away from the erect penis, it is impossible to maintain an erection. Imagine trying to fill a balloon with holes in it. As soon as the air is blown into the balloon, it leaks out. That is what happens in abnormal venous drainage. The condition is sometimes correctable by venous leak surgery, with the initial success rates ranging from fifty to sixty percent.

Unfortunately, the condition redevelops after a short time—usually in one or two years. Venous leak surgery is expensive, has many complications and is considered experimental by most authorities.

FAILURE TO FILL AND STORE

RADIATION THERAPY

Radiation therapy for cancer of the prostate, bladder, colon or testicle may cause scarring in the small penile blood vessels, making it difficult for the penis to fill and store blood. For example, over 50% of the men who have received radiation therapy for cancer of the prostate will notice a decrease of cessation of their erectile function as a side effect of the therapy.

DIABETES

Approximately 65% of the men who develop diabetes will become impotent within ten years. It is not uncommon for diabetes to be first diagnosed because the patient sought help for impotence. In our clinics, we often diagnose diabetes in unsuspecting individuals whose presenting complaint was impotence. Treatment and control of diabetes rarely reverses the impotence.

Diabetes is the major cause of impotence in young men in their twenties and thirties. Diabetes causes impotence in two ways. First, hardening of the arteries (arteriosclerosis) is accelerated resulting in restriction of blood flow to the penis. Second, nerve damage (neuropathy) prevents the normal transmission of nerve impulses to the blood vessels in the penis. This complication is a form of diabetic neuropathy, the same problem that causes loss of sensation or pain in the legs when those nerves are involved.

The impotent diabetic is normal in all other aspects of sexuality. He may have just as strong a sex drive as before his impotence. He simply is not able to get an erection. Like many other impotent men, diabetics can still be stimulated to ejaculation and orgasm even though the penis is soft. The impotence does not begin all at once—it is usually a slow decline in function.

As the diabetic's impotence advances, the nerve fibers are permanently damaged and the impotence becomes complete. Every young man developing signs of impotence should be tested for diabetes. Unfortunately, the problem cannot be reversed by simply controlling the diabetes, other measures are usually necessary.

HORMONAL CAUSES OF IMPOTENCE

The male hormone (Testosterone) is essential to the development of male sexual characteristics. However, a large amount of this circulating hormone need not be present for an erection to take place. It is well known that very young boys have very low testosterone levels, yet can still have erections. The male fetus even has erections inside his mother's uterus. Even castrated men, without testicles to provide testosterone, can occasionally get erections (although they usually report no desire to do so—I certainly can't blame them for that!)

The simple truth is that most men who are impotent have normal levels of testosterone. Even those with low testosterone usually have impotence from other causes. In most cases of impotence, administering testosterone is of little value, but it may give a man confidence, improving his performance for psychological rather than medical reasons. Certainly testosterone administration will improve sex drive (libido).

Small pituitary tumors may cause impotence by causing an increase in the hormone prolactin. Some studies have reported a high incidence of elevated prolactin levels in impotent men. Our experience has shown it to be exceedingly rare. If a high prolactin level is diagnosed, it can be reversed by administration of medication *Parlodel* (Bromocriptine).

DRUGS AND MEDICATION

Impotence can result as a side-effect of prescribed or over-the-counter drugs. There are over 200 commonly prescribed medications which can cause erectile problems, including alcohol and substance abuse.

ALCOHOL

In moderation, alcohol may be useful in sexual relations to repress inhibitions and increase socialization. Consuming too much, however, will depress the nervous system and create a numbing effect. Alcohol has an anesthetizing effect, so it isn't surprising that it is difficult to become aroused under its influence. Chronic alcohol abuse will generate a number of serious problems.

- Increase in estrogen levels—Estrogen is a female hormone which can work against the male hormone, testosterone, and reduce sexual desire. With alcohol abuse, the liver is damaged resulting in high estrogen levels.

- Peripheral neuropathy—A malfunction of the nerves to the penis may occur with prolonged alcohol abuse. Fifty percent of alcohol abusers who develop this neuropathy will continue to experience impotence even after they stop consuming alcohol.

- Decrease in testosterone—There may be a decrease in the male hormone, testosterone, due to the decrease of production in the testicles or breakdown of that hormone by the damaged liver. The testicles may even shrink in size.

One patient related, "I thought that drinking alcohol would relax me and help me to overcome my problem. Not knowing that alcohol made my impotence worse, I drank more. It was a vicious cycle! If I had only talked to a specialist first, I would have known that alcohol was not the answer."

MARIJUANA

By acting on the nervous system, marijuana can cause

depression of the male hormone, testosterone. Even though users report this drug intensifies orgasm, it can also inhibit normal erections and decrease sperm count. Cessation of use will reverse the drop in hormone levels.

Heroine, Cocaine, Crack, Amphetamines, Barbiturates, Sedatives, Tranquilizers, Sleeping Pills, Antihistamines, Antidepressants, and Phenothiazines are drugs that can act on the central nervous system and/or the peripheral nervous system. Any resulting interruption of the nerve impulse mechanism can cause impotence.

ULCER MEDICATIONS

Tagamet (Cimetidine) is a widely used drug for ulcer treatment. It can increase serum prolactin which may lead to lethargy, decreased sexual desire and physical impotence. Discontinued use of the medication corrects the condition. Zantac, an equivalent drug, does not cause prolactin problems and can often be substituted, but only with your physician's approval.

HIGH BLOOD PRESSURE MEDICATIONS

Prescription medications are high on the list of causes of impotence. Perhaps the most common impotency causing medications are those used to control high blood pressure. High blood pressure can be considered a medical condition where the heart pumps at a high pressure to supply blood through restricted blood vessels.

Many of the medications (anti-hypertensives) used to treat high blood pressure are linked to impotence. Listed below are some of the most commonly prescribed:

Generic Name	Brand Name
Spironolactone	Aldactazide, Aldatone
Methyldopa	Aldoclor, Aldoril, Aldomet
Clonidine Hydrochloride	Combipres, Catapres
Reserpine	Diupres, Regroton, Demi-Regroton, Aandril, Ser-Ap-Es, Salutensin Hydropres, Serpasil
Rauwolfia Serpentina	Raudixin, Harmonyl
Guanethidine Sulfate	Ismelin
Pargyline Hydrochloride	Eutonyl, Eutron
Chlorthalidone	Hygroton, Regroton, Combipres
Propranolol	Inderal

Sometimes, switching from one blood pressure medication to another will improve potency. Usually, however, the impotence is a result of vascular insufficiency and the elevated blood pressure is merely another manifestation of the same problem. In these cases, switching medications will be ineffective. *In our experience, the majority of impotent patients on anti-hypertensives will not benefit from changing medications.* The impotency seems more likely to be caused from restricted blood vessels than from the high blood pressure medication.

ESTROGEN THERAPY FOR CANCER OF THE PROSTATE

Estrogen therapy, which is sometimes used in the treatment of metastatic carcinoma of the prostate, will increase the level of this female hormone in the blood stream. Estrogen acts against the male hormone, testosterone. The patient will experience a decreased desire for sexual contact and a gradual loss of erectile function over a period of time.

IMPOTENCE AFTER SURGERY

With some surgeries, the nerves which achieve and maintain an erection may be injured. This is particularly common after colon, prostate, or bladder cancer operations. In removing the cancer completely, the adjacent nerves may be sacrificed. This damage compromises the ability to generate the proper nerve impulses to control erection.

The thought of cancer surgery is frightening for the average male. Because it is a life-threatening situation, he can be confused and under great emotional strain. Cancer surgery prompts the full range of emotions: fear, denial, withdrawal, anger, and depression. But despite the stress, quick decisions must be made to prevent further loss of health.

Many men will procrastinate when danger signs appear for fear of having cancer diagnosed. Waiting too long before visiting a doctor can only jeopardize life. Most medical problems have a solution—if diagnosed early.

Some men may delay seeking medical attention for fear of the possible impotence that can occur following cancer surgery. But, it's important to remember that cancer is life threatening; impotence, though serious, might alter your quality of life, but it won't cause you to die! Moreover, impotence is usually treatable by a competent urologist specializing in this dysfunction.

PEYRONIE'S DISEASE

Peyronie's Disease can be mistaken for cancer. A common symptom is a small lump which can be felt under the skin of the penis. The disease causes a scarring of the inside of the erectile compartments. As the scarring proceeds along the sides of the compartments, the penis becomes unable to remain straight during erection. The scar tissue begins to pull the penis to the side on which the scarring occurs, bending the penis toward the scar.

Sometimes the distortion of the penis is such that erection is painful or so crooked that penetration and successful intercourse are impossible. Worst of all, the blood flow to the penis may be restricted by the scarring, rendering the head of the penis floppy. This makes entry into the female vagina difficult or impossible. Peyronie's Disease is not uncommon in men ages forty to sixty-five. Its cause is unknown, but can be associated with excessive alcohol consumption.

Peyronie's Disease usually does maximum damage in the first two years and then becomes inactive, leaving the scar. There is no known cure. Medication, high doses of vitamins and injections with steroids have all been tried and have failed in extensive testing. Usually the scarring is not disabling but if impotence or severe curvature develops, surgery is needed.

Many operations have been devised but the best chance of success involves placement of a three-piece inflatable penile prosthesis. Surgery to remove the scarring without a penile implant shortens the penis (most men aren't in favor of that), and may make impotence worse.

PRIAPISM

Priapism is a painful, constant erection which occurs without sexual stimulation and persists beyond six hours. "Injection erection" programs as a treatment for impotence have made this rare condition relatively commonplace. It was formerly a problem only for patients with rare blood diseases such as sickle cell anemia. *Erection beyond 4 hours must be considered a medical emergency, and intervention by a urologist is necessary to prevent extensive scarring due to lack of blood flow and oxygen to the penis.*

Paradoxically, the usual end result of a bout of priapism is permanent failure to get an erection again. Impotence caused by priapism will require correction by the surgical implantation of a penile prosthesis.

IMPOTENCE CAUSED BY INJURY

Trauma to any portion of the pelvic region can cause

impotence. The *urogenital diaphragm* houses many fragile nerves and arteries which supply the penis. Severe injuries or fractures to the pelvis will break the nerves or interrupt the flow of blood to the penis.

Direct trauma to the penis can result in a fracture or rupture (aneurysm) of the erectile compartments. With this trauma, the patient experiences pain and swelling of the penis. No sexual activity is possible. This injury requires surgical correction. After repair, sexual function usually returns to normal.

Spinal cord trauma also causes impotence. The spinal cord is sheltered and protected by the neck and backbone (vertebral column). The vertebrae form a protective shield for the spinal cord. Injuries to the spinal cord may result in loss of the nerve center which controls erections. A person with this injury is unable to achieve erections through emotional stimulation. There are varying degrees of injuries to the spinal cord that can produce varying amounts of impotence.

A spinal cord injury dramatically changes the patient's lifestyle. Being confined to a wheelchair restricts the victim's vigorous, active life. If normal sexual relations can be continued, the emotional well-being of the patient and his partner may be preserved. Unfortunately, the majority of spinal cord injury patients lose the ability to get an erection at appropriate times.

Correction of this impotence can often preserve the family unit and correct the depression of being *less than a whole man*. This neurological impotence can be corrected by very small doses of medicine injected in the penis (injection erection) or a penile implant.

NEUROLOGICAL DISORDERS
when nerve fibers are damaged by disease

The control of blood flow into and out of the penis determines whether or not a man can have an erection. This control comes mainly from nerve fibers to the blood vessels. Stimulation of the penis sends impulses to the lower spinal cord and nerves from there send impulses which act to trap blood in the penis. Impulses from the brain may also run down the spinal cord to the blood vessels resulting in an erection (erotic thoughts will produce this).

There are numerous medical complications that may cause damage to the vital nerves that control erection. Impotence can occur with virtually any neurological disease. Some examples are neuropathy, chronic alcoholism, multiple sclerosis, muscular dystrophy, polio, surgery on neighboring structures or A.L.S. (Lou Gehrig's disease). The most common cause of neurological impotence, as we have mentioned earlier, is diabetes.

KIDNEY DISEASE

Since the kidneys act as the blood filtration system for the body, all medications, drugs, hormones and any other matter absorbed into the blood stream pass through the kidneys. When the kidneys are damaged and unable to perform this function, a man may become impotent because body waste products are allowed to pass back into the blood stream when they should be filtered and eliminated via the urine.

In the early 1960's, *kidney dialysis* was invented. With the use of the artificial kidney machine, all waste and excess water is filtered and removed from the patient. Unfortunately, many men on dialysis lose their ability to achieve erection because of emotional distress resulting from attachment to the dialysis machine. Other dialysis patients are rendered impotent from chemical changes in the body due to dialysis (e.g. lowering of male hormone in the blood.)

Kidney transplantation has fortunately become rather commonplace in the United States. After kidney transplantation, most patients report reversal of the impotence and resume normal sexual relations.

Chapter 4

Diagnosis of Impotence

Prior to 1974, physicians were taught that the cause of most impotence was "all in the mind." With the development of the inflatable penile prosthesis by the late F. Brantley Scott, M.D. and colleagues, medical researchers discovered that they had been doing a disservice to patients suffering from this disabling condition. Rather than impotence being a mental problem, doctors discovered that the usual cause was physical. Furthermore, a urologist who is trained to detect and treat impotence can discover the physical causes and reverse it in 95% or more of the cases!

Chronic impotence is a problem affecting millions of men in America, maybe as many as 20 million. As many as 90% of these men are unable to achieve erections because of *physical* reasons. The diagnosis and related treatment for physical impotence are usually covered by medical insurance and/or Medicare. Help is readily available for most impotent men no matter what the cause.

Almost all men, at one time or another, have had an incident of erectile failure. Occasional impotence can be provoked by a variety of causes such as anxiety, alcohol or fatigue. This temporary impotence will pass and does not require therapy. If the impotence persists over three months it can be considered chronic and medical help is needed.

Chronic impotence is the inability to achieve and maintain an erection over a prolonged period of time. Discounting any emotional, situational or short-term medical reason, a man should be able to recognize the symptoms of impotence by answering these questions:

CLUES TO PSYCHOLOGICAL IMPOTENCE

Answering "Yes" to any of these questions suggests your impotence may have a psychological basis.

- Do you have difficulty with premature ejaculation during sexual intercourse?

- Are you able to maintain an erection to complete sexual intercourse?

- Does it matter who your sexual partner is? Are you impotent with one and not with another?

- In the morning or the middle of the night, do you

experience full, sustained erections?

- Can you achieve full erection by touching or stroking the penis or through oral sex?

- If you masturbate, do you achieve normal erection?

- Have you recently experienced a break in a relationship with your primary sexual partner?

The reason a "yes" answer here *tends* to indicate a psychological basis is that if you answer yes, this very likely means that the erection mechanism is working, but that mentally you are shutting it down. In computer lingo you might say you have a *software* problem, not a hardware problem. Of course, as in some computers, recognize that things can go wrong with both at the same time.

CLUES TO PHYSICAL IMPOTENCE

Answering Yes to any of these questions points toward a physical cause for your erectile dysfunction.

- Can you achieve an erection but are unable to maintain it to complete sexual intercourse?

- Have you been diagnosed as diabetic? Have you ever been tested for diabetes? Does diabetes run in your family?

- In the past three months, have you failed to note an erection upon awakening in the middle of the night or when the alarm sounds?

- Do you take any medication which may cause impotence? (see Chapter 3)

- Did you become impotent after surgery?

- Have you observed any changes in the angle of the penis?

- Have you noticed any lumps or growths under the skin of the penis?

- Do you have any signs of hardening of the arteries?

- Are you over 60 years of age?

A "yes" answer questions tend to indicate a "hardware" problem; in other words, *the machine is just not working right.* Mentally, everything may be just fine. These are the kinds of problems we most often encounter.

During your medical evaluation, these and other questions may be asked. Your sexual and medical history represent the most important part of an impotence evaluation. In fact, some impotence experts are prepared to begin treatment with no other testing than a detailed history and physical. We find that most of the time, after asking some of these questions we have a pretty accurate idea what the primary problem is.

MIXED PHYSICAL/PSYCHOLOGICAL IMPOTENCE
When impotence has a physical cause but is magnified by chronic worry.

Impotence may be a variable problem in many patients. Sometimes they have trouble keeping the erection. Other times, there are problems getting the erection. These patients should not be consigned to the mental category automatically. Frequently, these patients have a contributing problem like early arteriosclerosis. This physical problem is then intensified severely by performance anxiety.

The patient is constantly thinking, "Will I make it?" No wonder he oftentimes becomes an emotional cripple. This mixed physical/psychological impotence is very common and almost always responsive to successful therapy. It is only necessary that the patient place himself in the hands of a competent urologist so that the problem can be properly evaluated and treated.

We see men who say they have problems with a spouse, but no problems with the secretary! Obviously this man probably does not need a urologist; we have a serious relationship problem here. It doesn't take long to figure out some problems, while others are quite complex.

TESTING FOR IMPOTENCE

It is important to note that while a wide range of tests are available to analyze various causes of impotency, the vast majority of patients do not require such extensive testing. After a complete history and physical examination, an impotence urologist can determine if *additional* tests are required. Many patients are treated in our clinics after a simple work-up consisting of NPT (Nocturnal Penile Tumescence) testing as discussed below. In some patients with obvious complete impotence, minimal evaluation may be needed and therapy is instituted on the first visit!

PHYSICAL EXAMINATION

A complete history and physical examination is the most important component of the urological work-up for impotence. Many times full testing is not needed for the impotence specialist to conclude what is the most likely problem. After the initial diagnosis, the patient can decide whether to have additional testing or to proceed with treatment. If additional testing is needed, the following tests are some which the patient may encounter.

NPT: NOCTURNAL PENILE TUMESCENCE MONITORING

Nocturnal Penile Tumescence (NPT) is a very accurate test used to indicate whether impotence is physical or psychological. A sleeping man normally has erections when he dreams. This dream state is called REM (rapid eye movement) sleep; it is an involuntary response. Normal erections occur one to five times a night and last between 20 and 30 minutes, and even longer. Think of all those wasted erections! If the cause of impotence is physical, the patient will not experience erections during REM sleep or the erections will be of poor quality.

Failure to generate nocturnal erections indicates a physical cause for the impotence. If good strong erections are recorded on NPT, psychological factors are more likely to be the actual cause of impotence. We see an occasional man who is not aware of any erectile activity, either awake or asleep, who then is shown to have perfectly normal erections during sleep. One gentleman recently seen was 44-years-old with his situation; *no known erections*. However, once measured with the equipment mentioned below, it turned out he had perfectly normal, 40-45 minute erections several times nightly. He was successfully treated with sex therapy methods.

Men who suffer physical impotence may achieve an erection but be unable to maintain that erection for a normal length of time. In addition, the erection may not be rigid enough for penetration of the female vagina. All these factors can be recorded and analyzed by the NPT if sophisticated machines such as *Dacomed Rigiscan* (see below) are utilized. Most authorities believe this test should be done over a two or three night period to increase accuracy. The NPT test has several forms.

SNAP-GAUGE TEST

The snap-gauge test is an NPT device which uses a soft band of material fitted around the penis and joined with velcro. Two or three threads of different lengths are attached to either side of the band to monitor erections and the strength of them. If the thread monitors are broken, a good erection has occurred during sleep for at least a few seconds. This test is inexpensive and performed in the patient's home.

Its disadvantage is that the results can be manipulated by the patient (by simply not wearing the snap-gauge). In addition, a broken gauge does not necessarily mean a *normal* erection, simply *some degree* of erection. Sometimes further testing may be needed. However, an unbroken snap-gauge is pretty good evidence of a physical basis for the impotence. Especially when combined with the patients' history and examination.

RIGIDITY AND TUMESCENCE MONITOR (DACOMED RIGISCAN)

The latest technology in NPT monitors is the *Rigidity and Tumescence monitor*. Gauges are placed around the base and near the tip of the penis. If an erection occurs, the expansion of the penis is measured by the strain gauge and recorded on a very small computer which the patient wears attached to his leg. This instrument measures the presence or absence of expansion of the penis as does the simple snap gauge.

More importantly, however, the Rigiscan quantifies the rigidity of the penis and measures the amount of time the erection is maintained. Expansion of the penis is measured at both base and tip of the penis. This test is performed in the patient's home and testing costs are usually covered by medical insurance.

Most authorities agree that a physician who specializes in impotence treatment should have a Rigiscan at his disposal. Just measuring the presence or absence of a change in penile circumference is sometimes not enough to assess true erectile dysfunction. The physician often needs information that only the Rigiscan can provide—whether true rigidity is attained and is constant for 10-20 minutes. Unfortunately, purchasing Rigiscan equipment is very costly (over $10,000) which often limits availability only to those urologists who treat a substantial amount of impotence.

Use of the Rigiscan also allows the impotence therapist to save time and money for the patient by using the rigidity information as a guide to selecting therapy. The degree of rigidity (penile plethysmography) shown by the Rigiscan indicates to the physician which therapy will have an excellent chance of success. Because the device measures rigidity, the urologist can often predict in advance whether injection therapy will be successful and whether low or high doses will be needed.

SLEEP LAB

Occasionally in medical-legal situations, a sleep lab is utilized to obtain even more accurate NPT and penile plethysmography readings. These labs are located in hospitals in large cities and the evaluation is quite expensive. The patient may be attached to an EEG to measure brain waves to determine if the correct level of sleep has been achieved. A nurse or an attendant will check for rigidity and firmness of the sleep erection, giving a numerical grade for evaluation purposes. Sometimes the attendant will awaken the patient for his evaluation of the erection. Surprisingly, the patient usually is more critical of the erection than the attendant.

BLOOD TESTS

Impotence can be caused by several metabolic and hormonal abnormalities. Diabetes, elevated cholesterol and testosterone deficiency are some of the most common causes. The testing of a patient with impotence (particularly a younger man) may include the following tests:

- *Blood sugar or glucose tolerance test*—to rule out the possibility of diabetes.

- *Prolactin hormone test*—Prolactin can be increased with the presence of a pituitary tumor or through the use of some medications such as Tagamet.

- *Serum testosterone test*—the male hormone which is important in sex drive. A great deficiency of this important hormone will result in a male with very little beard formation and small testicles. A small deficiency may cause poor erections.

- *Thyroid profile test*—This test measures thyroid activity. Low thyroid or hypothyroidism can be associated with erectile dysfunction.

Recognize that all men are different, and all situations are different, so your urologist may feel the need for more or less testing depending upon your particular problem. It would be difficult to call any particular test absolutely mandatory.

PENILE DOPPLER FLOW STUDIES

This is new, non-invasive technology done with sophisticated ultrasound machines to quantitate the ability of the penile blood vessels to respond to a demand for increased blood flow. This is accomplished by measuring the penile blood flow before and after penile injection with a drug to promote an erection, or at least increased blood flow within the penis.

Hardening of the arteries may compromise the ability of the vessels to expand resulting in a non-rigid (and thus incapable of penetration) erection. Similarly, veins that leak will cause a poor erection. Doppler flow tests will suggest these problems without the need for dye injection or X-rays as we will discuss below. For this reason, penile doppler flow studies have a great advantage over the more invasive tests listed below. These tests are basically painless and usually can be accomplished in about 30 minutes in the office. If the urologist does not have the equipment in the office, usually a local hospital will.

ARTERIOGRAPHY

To more accurately check the arterial blood supply of the penis, arteriography is performed. This test is accomplished by injecting dye into the main vessels supplying the penis and then following the dye's progress as it circulates in and through the penis. More accurate than the ultrasound explained above, it is also much more expensive and is not without complications. This test is generally reserved for very young patients with a history of some kind of trauma which may have injured the vessels of the penis.

It should be stressed that the vast majority of patients with vascular insufficiency show damage in the small vessels of the penis as a result of arteriosclerosis. These older individuals are not candidates for vascular repair. Elaborate testing and arteriography in these patients are not performed because the information that is derived has little or no clinical application.

CORPORA CAVERNOSOGRAM

This procedure involves a special X-ray study of the penis. The erectile chambers of the penis are injected with a dye and X-rays are taken. The study will diagnose venous leakage. *Cavernosography* is also helpful in diagnosing a patient with Peyronie's disease by showing constriction of the erectile chambers. Sometimes, pressure inside the penis during erection can be measured during this procedure.

BIOTHESIOMETRY

This is a very simple test to detect nerve impairment. The equipment generates a vibration and the patient is tested to detect his first sensation of feeling in the penis. If his first threshold is different from elsewhere in his body, nerve trouble is predicted and more sophisticated detection studies may be used. Impotent diabetics commonly have decreased penile sensation. This is not a commonly done test because usually the other tests are more practical, and offer more useful information.

NERVE STUDIES

Any neurogenic case of impotence can be studied through the use of a *bulbocavernosus reflex latency time study*. This series of tests measures the integrity of the nerve roots in the tailbone (sacrum). These nerve roots are important to erectile function. Electrodes are used to measure the time needed for nerve conduction to the penis. If the conduction is prolonged, this indicates a neurogenic cause for impotence. Generally speaking, this test does not usually have much clinical utility, and is not often done.

VASOACTIVE MEDICATION STIMULATION TEST

Papaverine, prostaglandin, or other drugs which cause penile arterial dilation and/or smooth muscle relaxation are injected into the penis and used for diagnostic evaluations.

The penis is injected and if an erection does not occur, either of the following problems are indicated:

- Significant obstruction of arteries feeding the penis, or,

- Severe vein leakage so that blood cannot be maintained in the erectile chambers.

If the circulatory problem is not too severe, papaverine, phentolamine, prostaglandin E1 or other agents may overcome mild to moderate circulatory or *vasculogenic* impotence and thus be used as a therapy. Since the injections of these *vasoactive* drugs bypass the peripheral nerves and the central nervous system, it can be a useful way to gain information suggesting psychogenic impotence or peripheral neuropathy (nerve damage.) Papaverine and other "injection erection" agents have been excellent tools in the diagnosis of impotence. In Chapter 6 we will discuss, in depth, the use of these agents as a treatment for impotence.

CASE STUDY

Roland was only 33-years-old when he sought relief from impotence after admittingly having this problem for as long as he could remember. He had been married two years, and the erection failure was causing stress. His wife was worried that he had another lover. He was tormented by his problem, and was *desperate* for help. To cut-to-the-chase, he's okay now, and he and his wife are both very happy.

All it took to rectify Roland's problem was a fairly advanced evaluation, along with his history and examination and some blood work, all of which was normal. The Rigiscan testing revealed poor nocturnal erections, just as we expected with this history. In this particular situation a decision was made to further study the circulation of the penis, which demonstrated "venous leak". Blood was getting into the penis properly, but was leaving much too quickly, so a true erection could not occur.

After a lot of discussion about alternatives, he is presently functioning fairly well with a vacuum constriction device. It is a great relief to him (and to his wife) to understand the problem. He has found the vacuum device a little cumbersome, and will probably undergo penile prosthesis surgery in the near future.

This was a fairly complicated situation, and more than the usual amount of testing was necessary to arrive at a satisfactory diagnosis and outcome. Fortunately, most patients have much more straightforward problems, requiring considerably less evaluation.

Chapter 5

Impotency Treatments Infrequently Utilized

A book devoted to impotence therapy would not be complete without discussion of the following treatments. However, the reader should remember that these therapies are infrequently utilized and we direct you to Chapter 6 for discussion of more common impotency treatments.

Once the urologist has determined whether the impotence is physical or psychological, they can recommend treatment. If, by the use of the *Nocturnal Penile Tumescence Test*, the urologist determines that the physical mechanism is intact, it is the urologist's responsibility to direct his patients to the appropriate mental health professional that will offer the best treatment for their psychological problem. Often, the best results are achieved when the urologist and the mental health professional work together in finding the proper treatment.

PSYCHOLOGICAL COUNSELING AND THERAPY

If the cause of impotence is psychological, a psychiatrist, psychologist or sexual counselor specializing in impotency should be contacted. Counseling and therapy should begin as soon as possible to get the patient back to sexual function.

There are many different aspects of successful psychological treatment. The primary goal of counseling is to reduce the stress and anxiety associated with performance. There may also be other emotional difficulties to overcome.

Communication and openness are imperative to successful psychological therapy. It is up to the therapist to decide whether the counseling sessions are honest and straightforward. Stress at work or at home could be aggravating the situation. Other obstacles could include intense religious beliefs or personal inhibitions.

When total honestly is determined, the counselor may instruct the couple in natural sexual behavior skills. Guiding the couple step-by-step and teaching relaxation techniques help diminish anxiety and build up self-esteem. This instruction also helps strengthen the emotional ties between the couple, allowing them to become more intimate and to share with one another and the counselor during therapy.

COUNSELING AND THERAPY METHODS

- *Sensate Focusing*—Hugging, massaging and kissing the

hands, neck and face, or whatever is comfortable to the partner, in non-threatening situations should cause the erection naturally.

- *The Seductive Mode*—Instruction begins with the patients' clothes on and slowly progresses to removal several hours later.

- *The Erection Mode*—During the sensate focusing and seduction mode therapies, firm erections may develop. However, the patient may need to have his partner fondle his genitalia to improve erection. The patient must then be counseled not to use it instantaneously.

- *Hypnotherapy*—While under hypnosis, subconscious messages are given to the patient in order to help him achieve a good erection.

- *Surrogate Counseling*—For the single man who does not have a partner, a surrogate sexual partner is recommended to help in practicing the exercises. This should only be done under the supervision of a qualified professional.

The psychological sex counseling program promotes education, counseling techniques and homework assignments that reinforce what is learned in the more formal counseling sessions.

There are many factors which may inhibit the success of psychological therapy. Interpersonal dynamics, lack of time, lack of patience, or lack of funds may spell failure for psychotherapy as a solution for psychological impotence. Most studies list the success rate for sexual counseling at less than 50%.

If, after an adequate trial of sexual counseling, the patient is still suffering from erectile problems, many urologists will institute one of the treatments outlined in the next chapter usually a vacuum erection device or "injection erection." In rare instances the urologist may implant a penile prosthesis for these troubling cases.

MEDICAL TREATMENTS FOR IMPOTENCE

YOHIMBINE

Once considered by the ancient Greeks as an aphrodisiac, this medication, derived from the bark of a tree, improves penile blood flow by causing restriction of outflow of blood from the penis. It may also have a central effect in the brain to increase sex drive (libido). For this reason some physicians have treated female frigidity with this drug. The drug is well tolerated, has few side effects and is relatively inexpensive about ($25.00 for 30 days).

In the past, yohimbine has been combined with various other drugs to form a kind of "impotence cocktail" in the vehicle of a single capsule. Some of the drugs used include *strychnine, caffeine, testosterone, zinc* and even *amphetamines*. There is no evidence that these combination capsules worked better than yohimbine alone in adequate doses.

Yohimbine is sold in health food stores and over the counter without a prescription but the dosages are inadequate for effectiveness. The usual dosage for the prescription drug is 5.4 mg. three times per day, although some doctors suggest increasing to as much as 43 mg. per day. If the divided dosage is ineffective, we have found 16.2 mg. (three pills) prior to intercourse occasionally successful. At least two weeks of therapy is necessary prior to evaluating the success or failure of therapy. When yohimbine works, the therapy must usually be continued indefinitely or the impotence is likely to return.

Medical literature reports approximately a 25% success rate with yohimbine in physically impotent men. It seems to work least well in cases of vascular insufficiency. In our experience, the probability of success can be predicted by the results of the penile rigidity and duration of erection information (penile plethysmography) obtained from nocturnal tumescence testing with the *Dacomed Rigiscan.*

The response rate of physically impotent men to yohimbine is at best marginal. Nevertheless, because of ease of administration, safety and modest cost, the drug is frequently tried in patients as a first line of therapy. Many patients initially will not accept more invasive methods and want to solve their problem with a "magic pill." Prescribing yohimbine first often helps them to see that oral drugs won't provide the answer and prepares them to accept other treatments. Side effects, while infrequent, are anxiety, nausea, flushing and dizziness.

CORRECTING HORMONE IMBALANCE OF
PROLACTIN AND TESTOSTERONE

High levels of *prolactin* (the hormone secreted from the pituitary gland which stimulates the testicle to make testosterone) can cause impotence in men without any other symptoms. This may very rarely be related to a pituitary tumor but more often is due to medication or to hormonal imbalance. The overproduction of prolactin may be corrected by administration of the drug *Parlodel* (bromocriptine). High levels of prolactin are found in less than 1% of all men seen with impotence.

Low levels of testosterone may rarely be due to hormonal imbalance. Usually, however, low testosterone levels are due to unknown causes. After diseases of the pituitary gland, testicles and thyroid are ruled out, the low testosterone level can be treated by injection administration of 100-300 mg. of long-acting hormone every three or four weeks. If the patient's impotence is due to this cause it should rapidly reverse in a dramatic fashion.

Unfortunately, our experience is that impotence is rarely caused by low testosterone and most impotent patients do not benefit from hormone supplementation. Worst of all, testosterone injections may leave the patient with increased desire (libido) but still without the ability to generate a decent erection!

Most authorities consider oral testosterone a waste of time and money since the hormone is poorly absorbed in the gastrointestinal tract. For testosterone to work effectively it must be given by injection or by patch application.

Patients who do receive testosterone should be closely monitored for the development of prostate cancer. The injections do not seem to cause prostate cancer, but if it develops, the supplemental testosterone encourages the cancer's growth.

STOP SMOKING

Vasoconstriction is narrowing of the penile blood vessels, and is caused by nicotine in tobacco resulting in decreased blood flow to the penis. Prolonged smoking over many years also increases deposition of material called colloid in the walls of the small vessels of the penis which is a direct cause of "failure to fill" impotence.

Authorities estimate that "50 pack years" are necessary to cause impotence. Pack years are defined as the number of packs smoked daily times years smoked. For example, a man 50 years old who had been smoking 2 packs daily for 32 years would be described as having 64 pack years.

Stopping smoking may improve erections. If the individual uses the new popular patches such as *Nicoderm* or *Habitrol* as an aid to stopping smoking, no effect will be noted until the patches have also been stopped since they contain nicotine. Some medical studies show the drug *Isoxsuprine* has been effective in returning erections in patients who have been heavy smokers and quit. The dosage is 10-20 mg daily and unpleasant side effects are rare.

Unfortunately, older individuals who usually have assoc-ated arteriosclerosis, may have irreversible damage, and smoking cessation will not return potency. In our practice, however, smoking cessation is requested of the patient even though the potency restoring results are unencouraging. In our view, there are many, many other smoking-related health-problems which are much more threatening to ones existence than impotence. We view impotence therapy as a good opportunity to help the patient eliminate this self-destructive addiction.

REDUCING ALCOHOL CONSUMPTION

In small amounts, alcohol may be a social lubricant and a sexual facilitator. One or two cocktails, beers or glasses of wine may actually enhance the ability to get an erection. More than one or two, however, acts as a depressant and may inhibit erection. Alcohol abuse acts as anesthesia and positively prevents erection. The temporary lack of the ability to get an erection after a night of hard drinking is well known to heavy drinkers. The impotence may even carry over until the next morning. Inability to orgasm is another effect of heavy indulgence and may persist for twenty-four hours.

Abuse of alcohol over long periods (alcoholism) leads to nerve and liver damage and may result in permanent impotence. Alcoholics develop *peripheral neuropathy,* a condition which results in the small nerves which are the farthest from the central nervous system being damaged. The symptoms are spotty lack of sensation, trouble telling the position of ones feet, and trouble with coordination of complicated small movements. Alcoholics also develop damage to the small nerves which regulate erection.

The liver damage sustained by long term alcohol abuse

causes hormone imbalance with an overproduction of the female hormone, *estrogen*, and an underproduction of the male hormone, testosterone.

Alcoholics frequently have very little interest in sexual activity when in love with the bottle. After treatment, the recovered alcoholic may frustratingly find that he is unable to get an erection even though he has been alcohol-free for several years. His long history of alcohol abuse has damaged his nerves permanently. *In our experience, a period of alcohol abuse as a young man may cause impotence from other causes to appear at a much earlier age even though alcohol abuse has not been present for many years.*

Heavy smoking and heavy drinking are high-risk factors for the onset of impotence at a relatively early age. We see a large number of patients with impotence in their early 50's who were—or are—heavy smokers and drinkers. These men have no other demonstrable causes for their impotence but are physically impotent when tested with the nocturnal tumescence test. *The combination of alcohol and nicotine abuse is a particularly potent precipitator of failure in the bedroom.*

VASCULAR (ARTERIAL BYPASS) SURGERY

Normal erection depends upon a 7-fold increase in arterial blood flow. Obviously, patients with significant generalized arterial disease or localized penile arterial problems will not be able to provide an adequate increase in arterial inflow after appropriate nerve messages are received by the blood vessels. Vascular corrective surgery on the penis utilizing arterial bypass (similar to heart bypass) is done in a few centers in the United States and Europe.

Patients with significant risk-factors such as heart attack, high blood pressure, prolonged cigarette smoking, high cholesterol or age older than 50 are generally not candidates for vascular corrective surgery. Young patients with localized arterial problems from an injury may have excellent results from vascular bypass surgery in the penis. This is similar to the procedure commonly done in the coronary arteries. In a group of highly selected patients the success rate can be as high as 60%. The surgery is very time consuming, expensive, and has significant side effects of penile swelling and possible lack of penile sensation.

VASCULAR (VENOUS LEAK) SURGERY

Another type of vascular surgery can be performed for some young patients who initially have very good erections that diminish quickly prior to completion of intercourse. When these patients are studied with cavernosography, abnormal veins and abnormal drainage of blood can be documented. These patients are called "venous leakers".

Surgery has been developed to close off these abnormal drainage channels, and in properly selected patients the initial success rate can be as high as 60%. Unfortunately, the percentage of happy patients diminishes with time, and after two years, less than 40% of the patients report satisfactory erections. Like arterial surgery the venous leak surgery is expensive, time consuming and may be associated with unpleasant side effects such as swollen penis and sensation problems. *Keep in mind, there are very few men who even might benefit from this specialized surgery.*

Although *revascularization surgery* of arteries and veins of the penis cannot boast the greater than 95% patient-partner satisfaction of penile implants, newly impotent men continue to desire restoration of erection naturally if possible. This will continue to stimulate research in new methods of vascular surgery and new chemical agents. *As of this writing, less than 1% of all patients with impotence are truly candidates for vascular reconstruction.*

Chapter 6

Common Impotency Treatments

In the previous chapter, we discussed various treatments which are only *occasionally* used or are usually unsuccessful. Let us now turn our attention to the treatment methods *most commonly used* in America.

- Vacuum Constriction Devices
- Penile Injection Therapy
- Penile Prosthetic Implants

These are the three therapies utilized on over 90% of all American impotence patients treated. We'll analyze each of these methods in a critical fashion, breaking each treatment down into positive and negative aspects.

VACUUM RESTRICTION DEVICE

The Vacuum Restriction Device comes under several brand names such as: *Response, Touch, ErecAid,* and *VED.* External Vacuum Therapy is a mechanical, nonsurgical method of filling the penis with blood and simulating a natural erection. It is based on the principle that an erection can be produced by placing the penis in a vacuum chamber or cylinder which promotes blood flow into the erectile tissue of the penis.

Air is removed from the cylinder by a pump (manual or electric), drawing blood into the penis. The erection is maintained by trapping the blood in the penis with the application of a tight elastic band around the base of the penis. After the tension ring is placed around the base of the penis the vacuum chamber is removed (see Fig.3). The patient may then proceed with intercourse. The rubber band may be left in place up to 30 minutes.

External vacuum devices have been used in thousands of patients. Some are happy with the devices as a long-term management of erection inadequacy. They are also useful as a temporary aid during counseling for psychological impotence. Some urologists use these devices as an aid in determining the true interest of patients considering penile implant surgery.

Some European doctors have reported improved natural erections after vacuum therapy but this is unsubstantiated in American medical literature. Extremely few serious injuries have been reported with these devices, although bruising is common.

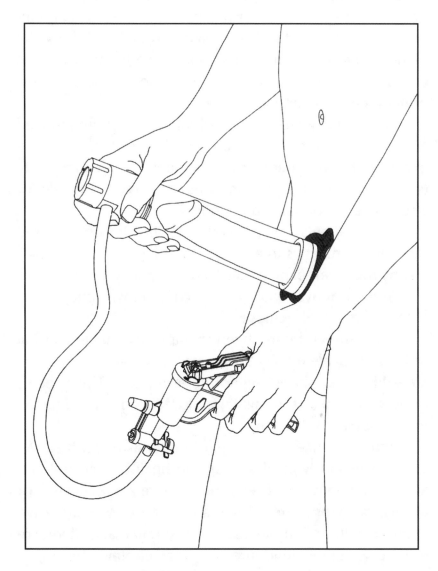

Figure 3 - "Vacuum Constriction Device"

In our experience, vacuum therapy has a *very high drop-out rate*. A survey of our patients showed that after one year only one-third were satisfied and still using the device. The remainder had either converted to "injection erection" therapy or "penile implantation" or lost interest in impotence therapy altogether.

Our patients were concerned that the vacuum induced erection was cold, blue, numb and floppy. This can be explained because one-third of the penis is within the body (see Fig.9) and this portion is not engorged with blood. Thus the erection has no anchor.

Other patients complained that the device required seven to ten minutes to activate, foreplay was interrupted, and by then their partner was "out of the mood." Additionally, if the ring was too tight, ejaculation was uncomfortable or difficult to achieve.

There are at least fifteen companies manufacturing devices available by physician prescription and many more are sold in "sex shops" without prescription. There seems to be great interest in this type of treatment by the newly impotent patient.

Vacuum devices have much to offer as initial therapy. They are relatively painless, have no significant side effects and are non-invasive. They don't require a needle-stick or a surgical procedure. They are relatively inexpensive ($250-$550), and in most states, insurance and Medicare reimburses the expenditure to a degree. Nevertheless, in our experience, most persons seriously interested in resuming a natural sex life only spend a brief period of time with this therapy.

PENILE INJECTION THERAPY— "INJECTION ERECTION"

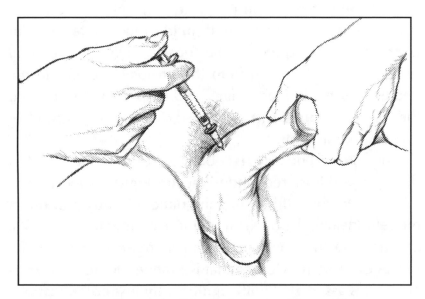

Figure 4 - "Penile Injection Therapy"

One of the most popular methods of treating impotence involves the injection of a small amount of medication directly into the penile erectile tissue. The medication dilates arteries and relaxes the delicate smooth muscle of the erectile chambers. Overall blood flow through the penis is facilitated and the erection is natural and rigid. The medication is injected directly into the corpora cavernosa with a tiny needle with only a pinch of discomfort. Erection usually occurs within 10-15 minutes and unlike that induced by the vacuum device, is very similar to a natural erection. The erection typically lasts 30 to 90 minutes.

Sixty-five percent of all impotent patients respond favorably to injection therapy. It is particularly useful in *neurogenic impotence* (e.g. spinal cord injury). These patients often require only tiny amounts of medication. It is also helpful in patients with mild to moderate vascular impotence but requires higher doses. *Rigiscan nocturnal tumescence testing* can help the urologist quantitate the degree of erectile inadequacy and help plan dosage, and the *duplex doppler ultrasound studies* are very useful in this manner as well.

The proper dosage is obtained by a series of test dosages administered under the urologist's supervision. While undergoing this testing the patient is taught to inject himself. Ideally, the medication induced erection is a 75% erection, so that the patient can increase it to 100% by sexual excitement. Dosage that is planned to achieve 75% erection is associated with significantly less complications than injecting enough to give a full (100%) erection without sexual excitement.

There are several drugs available for "injection erection." *Papaverine*, a vasodilator developed for coronary vessels, was the first to be used in 1984. Later *phentolamine* was added to facilitate the papaverine and allow lowering of the dosage needed. The mixture of these drugs has allowed thousands of men to return to a healthy sex life. Unfortunately, large series of injection patients using these two drugs reported a complication rate as high as 20%.

The most frequent problem was the development of

priapism, the occurrence of a prolonged erection in the absence of sexual excitement. These chemically induced erections simply will not go away! The blood sludges in the penis and requires detoxification of the chemical causing the erection. The patient must report to the emergency room, usually in the middle of the night, and antidotes to the "injection erection" must be injected into the penis to counteract the erection.

Occasionally it is necessary for the urologist to use large needles to withdraw the sludged blood. Rarely, surgery is necessary to reverse the erection. *Erection lasting longer than four hours should be considered a medical emergency and the patient must arrange for detoxification.* The problem of priapism after "injection erection" is annoying but reversible, if treated promptly. It can be disastrous if treatment is delayed many hours. *The end result of untreated priapism is a scarred penis incapable of any future erection!*

Another problem associated with injection therapy is bruising at the site of injection. A more serious complication of injection therapy is the development of scar tissue (fibrosis) on the inside of the corporal body at the site of the injection. This may cause shortening and crookedness of the penis much like the crookedness seen in Peyronie's disease.

It is also recognized that many men develop tolerance to the medication, thus requiring increasingly higher doses over time. High doses increase the likelihood that complications may occur. Eventually, despite high doses, the medication is no longer useful. Most men (needless to say) hesitate and think hard (no pun intended) on this procedure. But wait, there are better methods to try. It is noteworthy that recently, the manufacturer of papaverine, Eli Lilly, has to a large extent withdrawn the drug from the market for this use, so it is harder to obtain. And, many urologists have ceased using this particular drug. There are some other options however.

In the late 1980's a new injectable medication became available, *prostaglandin E1* (PGE-1). This hormone-like substance produces the same acceptable erection but has a significantly lower incidence of priapism. Unfortunately, the medication is quite expensive and current costs show an injection of prostaglandin E1 sufficient to cause an erection will cost between $10 and $20. Another disadvantage of this new medication is that it deteriorates if kept at room temperature for any length of time. Even refrigerated, PGE-1 will only remain effective for four to six months.

Finally, many patients complain of mild pain at the injection site lasting an hour or two. Sometimes this pain can be eliminated by allowing the medication to warm up to room temperature prior to injection rather than self-injecting medication taken directly from the refrigerator.

In the previous edition of this book, we sang the praises of a mixture of *Papaverine, Phentolamine and PGE-1*. This "cocktail" or "triple mix" of the three drugs allowed each drug dosage to be reduced so that cost was lowered, but effectiveness was raised.

Unfortunately, as we noted above, in December, 1994, Eli Lilly, the manufacturer of Papaverine, ceased to produce the drug due to the fear of lawsuits. Some Papaverine available now is from foreign countries and we consider it to be, perhaps, less reliable. Many urologists have ceased to prescribe the "triple mix" out of fear of the unpredictability of the generic Papaverine and many other urologists have followed suit.

The good news, however, is that in July of 1995 the FDA approved Prostaglandin for injection into the penis under the trade namet *Caverje*. It has been available commercially for some time in Britain and other European countries. Although at this time we do not have cost figures, it is probably in the $15 to $30 per erection range, depending on the dose required. With FDA approval, PGE-1 should experience greater success in the USA, as many patients have deferred injection therapy because of fear of complications, fueled by the FDA's reluctance to approve its use.

Despite the hope of PGE's continued good safety record and recent FDA approval, the bad news is that PGE-1 is not often as effective as the old "triple mix."It simply does not work on as many impotent patients and is least effective on patients with significant vascular insufficiency. Older patients, with the onset of impotence in their late 50's to 70's, frequently have slowly progressive arteriosclerosis or hardening of the arteries. These men frequently will not respond to PGE-1. In addition, for the man who does initially respond to PGE-1, it may later lose its effectiveness as the hardening of the arteries continues to progress or as his body becomes tolerant to the medication.

As long as only one of these drugs is approved by the FDA, many urologists are reluctant to prescribe "injection erection" therapy out of a fear of malpractice action. Many impotence specialists require the patient to sign an "informed consent" release prior to embarking on an injection program. This, perhaps, is an overreaction since PGE-1 has such a well-demonstrated safety record.

Despite these negative factors, tens of thousands of men nationwide (hundreds in our practices alone) are involved in "injection erection" programs. Many of these men are very happy with the resumption of sexual activity and willing to undergo the minimal risk. Our current survey shows that 50% of our injection patients are very satisfied with their therapy after one year versus 33% of vacuum device and 95% of inflatable implant patients.

In our view, injection therapy is appropriate as a *primary therapy* if the patient is fully informed about the risks. It is also useful for those men who are considering a prosthesis implant but are hesitant to go through a surgical procedure, or patients who do not have the financial resources for prosthesis implantation. We sometimes use an injection of vasoactive material in our diagnostic work-up and utilize the resultant erection (or lack of) to counsel the patient as to how seriously he should consider surgical implantation.

While many impotency centers use *injection therapy* as their most common form of therapy, we continue to consider it, at present, short term therapy. This view could change with the development of better injection agents.

We worry a bit about using injection therapy in the younger man, because the idea of sticking needles into the penis for many years can certainly lead to fibrosis (scarring) and most likely, the more injections a person has, the greater the likelihood of these problems. If you are considering this type of therapy, keep these things in mind.

PENILE PROSTHESIS IMPLANTS

A penile prosthesis is a device which is surgically implanted within the penis and allows the impotent man to obtain an erection upon demand. Currently there are three types of penile implants; the malleable, the self-contained inflatable, and the multiple component inflatable. Some of the older models had problems but the new ones are more dependable. Research continues, and each edition of this book may be slightly incomplete in this area because of these newer developments.

Today, penile implantation is a very safe procedure and the prostheses are relatively complication-free. In fact, we are currently experiencing a five year success rate of 86% for all types of prostheses combined. That means that only 14% of all the implants have some kind of difficulty which requires re-operation in the first five years. If we look at re-operation required by mechanical problems, the 5 year success rate is approaching 96%. It was not always so. In fact, in the 1970's the devices had as high as 70% revision rate, usually for mechanical reasons. This statistic initially gave prosthetic surgery as a treatment for impotence a tarnished reputation among many urologists.

HISTORY OF THE PENILE PROSTHESIS

The first penile implant was performed in 1936 when a surgeon took a piece of rib cartilage and implanted it in a man's penis as a stiffening device. It was eventually absorbed by the body and stopped working. However, this report stimulated research and many subsequent attempts to find a material which would stiffen the impotent penis and allow penetration.

In 1972, Drs. Small and Carrion at the University of Miami invented the semi-rigid malleable rod. These flexible rods were implanted in the penile corporal bodies. The rods were molded from medical grade silicone and were well tolerated by the patients. Furthermore, the patients reported functional success.

In 1973, the late Dr. F. Brantley Scott of Baylor College of Medicine in Houston, was instrumental in the invention of the first inflatable penile prosthesis. This was a major advancement and allowed the patient to have command over when he wished an erection and when he wished softness (flaccidity). This inflatable device was remarkable since it was undetectable in the soft state and the erection was quite natural. All the devices listed below are further improvements of the designs invented by these innovative urologists.

MALLEABLE IMPLANT, SEMI-RIGID STYLE
Brand Names: *Small-Carrion, Mentor Malleable, Mentor Accuform, AMS 600, Jonas, Subrini*

This semi-rigid implant has been used by physicians for over twenty years. During these two decades many different versions have been developed. This style of implant creates a permanent semi-erection and, depending on the implant used, offers varying degrees of concealment. These implants are technically the easiest to implant, are the least expensive, and have a very low rate of mechanical complication. The big disadvantage is that the erection is not as good as that created by an inflatable model. It is not as rigid and lacks girth expansion when compared to the inflatable models. Another major disadvantage is that the penis is always semi-hard, and therefore may be difficult to conceal, causing social embarrassment.

More recently, semi-rigid rods have incorporated a hinge or wire core as an aid to concealment. These devices allow the patient to bend the penis down or up, depending upon need. While an improvement over the original semi-rigid rods (Small-Carrion, Jonas), our patients still report the need to adjust the penis when changing body positions such as from sitting to standing or vice-versa.

Experience with these prostheses over the past 20 years has shown us that mechanical dependability for the long term has been very good. Medical complications, however, may be more common than with inflatable implants. The stiffness of the rods over time causes weakening in the corpora cavernosa with resultant erosion of the components through the skin. For this reason they often should not be used in spinal cord injury patients and diabetics.

Another problem we have noted is that the rods act as tissue expanders lengthening the penis a small amount. After this happens, what was formerly an adequate erection becomes floppy causing patient dissatisfaction. Due to the availability of other superior prosthesis designs, we find that not too many of our patients choose these malleable implants.

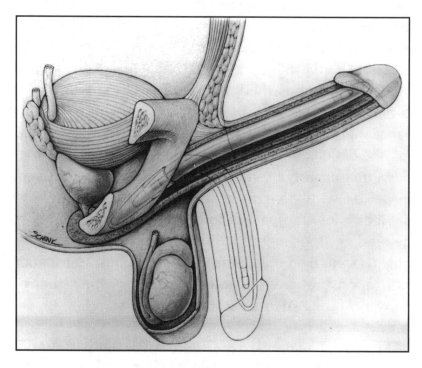

Figure 5 - "Malleable Prosthesis, Semi Rigid Style"

MALLEABLE IMPLANT—POSITIONABLE STYLE
Brand Name: *Dacomed Omniphase*

This prosthesis is the most technically advanced of the malleable devices. It consists of a series of small plastic blocks strung together on a steel cable like a string of pearls. It is implanted in the same simple fashion as a semi-rigid rod. When the patient bends the penis to the erect position, a spring mechanism tightens the cable and pulls the blocks together in an interlocked position which produces rigidity of the penis. When the penis is bent down, the cable is released, blocks separate, and considerable softness is achieved.

This device has advantages over other non-inflatable devices. It is fairly easy for the surgeon to implant and it is more concealable than most of all the non-inflatable devices. The disadvantages are that it is almost as expensive as an inflatable penile prosthesis and the erection is not as satisfactory. The device is also quite noticeable upon handling the penis.

SELF-CONTAINED INFLATABLE PENILE IMPLANT
Brand Name: *Dynaflex*

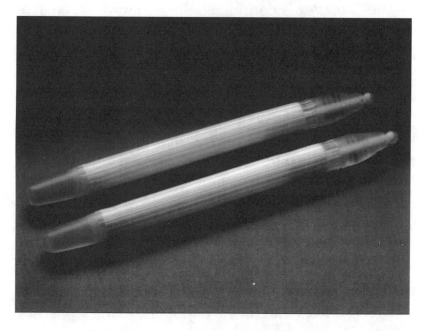

Figure 6 - "Self-Contained Inflatable Prosthesis: Dynaflex"

This self-contained inflatable implant is surgically placed through a tiny incision at the base of the penis. There is only one such device remaining in the marketplace, the *Dynaflex* manufactured by American Medical Systems. This prosthesis can be considered a "liquid rod."

The system contains a reservoir filled with fluid, valves and inflation pump—all within a single implantable unit. Erection is achieved by squeezing the pump located behind the head of the penis. Two prosthetic devices are necessary, one for each corporal body. Thus, it is necessary to pump each prosthesis several times to achieve the erection. Deflation is achieved by bending the penis 90 degrees and holding the bend for 10 seconds. This activates a release valve, fluid flows back into the reservoir, and the penis becomes soft.

The *Dynaflex* is considered the easiest of all inflatable devices to implant and is sometimes accompanied by less patient discomfort following surgery than the multi-component inflatable implants. The surgery causes so little discomfort that the operation can usually be done as an outpatient, and even under local anesthetic for some men. While truly an inflatable device, flaccidity (softness) is not completely attainable, as the penis maintains semi-rigidity.

Erection is also not optimum because there is little girth expansion. When compared to the three-piece implants (described below), both flaccidity and erection are not as satisfying. Nevertheless, the results with a self-contained implant are superior to the malleable and positionable prostheses covered in preceding sections.

The *Dynaflex* has been a popular choice for older patients who want the least amount of surgery and want a dependable, readily concealable device. It is less important to these individuals how the prosthesis looks when either erect or soft. Dr. Wilson, one of the authors of this book, participated in the clinical investigation of these devices when they were under review for the FDA. After approval we were very enthusiastic and implanted almost 300 Dynaflexes and its "older brother" the Hydroflex.

Unfortunately, experience has shown us that the semi-rigidness of these devices acts as a *tissue expander* over time causing a slight lengthening of the penis. This results in the development of a floppy erection after two years and results in many unsatisfied patients. We have removed some of the self-contained implants for either mechanical breakdown or patient dissatisfaction.

We usually replaced the prostheses with three-piece inflatable implants and most patients were much happier with their new erections. Our experience has shown us that the three-piece inflatable implant offers superior mechanical reliability and higher patient satisfaction. Presently, there is very little reason to utilize self-contained inflatables.

THE DYNAFLEX AS TREATMENT FOR PREPUBIC RECESSION
The Disappearing Penis

Some older, overweight patients have a condition doctors call *prepubic recession* of the penis. This condition, due to obesity and poor muscle tone, is characterized by a man whose penis appears to have receded into his body. Some people call this the "disappearing penis." The *Dynaflex* is sometimes the prosthesis of choice for these men since the relative rigidity of the device brings the penis outside the plane of the body, giving a good cosmetic appearance both in flaccidity and erection.

We have treated the problem of prepubic recession with great success by use of a *Dynaflex* implant. But because the three-piece inflatable offers improved mechanical reliability and higher patient satisfaction, we generally prefer the three-piece for most patients and recommend the *Dynaflex* for certain situations. It is also useful in a situation where a man has had extensive abdominal surgery making placement of a reservoir of the three-piece prosthesis difficult and even technically impossible. Your urologist will be the best person to make these types of decisions with you, because each patient and each situation is a little different.

MULTI-COMPONENT INFLATABLE, TWO PIECE
Brand Name: *Ambicor*

Early in 1995, American Medical Systems introduced an improved Dynaflex called the Ambicor. This prosthesis combines the standard Dynaflex cylinders with a tiny scrotal pump which makes the prosthesis easier to inflate than pumping the tips of the Dynaflex cylinders individually. Deflation is accomplished by flexing the prosthesis for 10-15 seconds as in the standard Dynaflex.

Our very limited experience with this prosthesis, coupled with an extensive history with the Dynaflex, leads us to believe this prosthesis will be inferior to the three-piece inflatables in both mechanical reliability and patient satisfaction. Since the cylinders are the same as the old Dynaflex, we predict decreased quality of erection after two years and mechanical unreliability after five. We will closely monitor the success of this prosthesis.

Dr. Mobley, one of the authors of this book, was involved in the investigative development of this prosthesis and has had so far, fairly extensive, successful outcomes.

MULTI-COMPONENT INFLATABLE, TWO-PIECE
Brand Name: *Mentor Mark II*

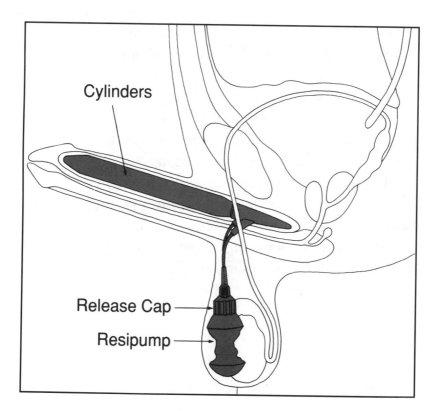

Figure 7 -" Two-Piece Inflatable Prosthesis: Mentor Mark II"

This variation of the classic inflatable implant is manu-factured by Mentor Corporation who also makes an excellent three-piece inflatable *Mentor Alpha I* prosthesis discussed below. In an effort to market a device which does not require an abdominally positioned reservoir, this implant combines pump and reservoir in a single unit which resides in the scrotum. The second part of the device contains preconnected cylinders placed in the penis.

The Mark II produces satisfactory erection and flaccidity and requires less surgery to implant than the three-piece devices outlined below. It's primarily used in those cases where the urologist wishes to avoid placing a reservoir in the abdomen. This may be the case in patients who are quite obese, or who have had extensive radiation or abdominal surgery. The disadvantage of this implant is that the scrotal reservoir has the capability of delivering only one-half ounce (15cc) of fluid to the cylinders.

After a period of time, this may not be enough fluid for a firm erection. The manufacturer advises that the device can have more fluid added by injecting the system through the skin but this has the theoretical chance of causing an infection. In our experience, some of the implanted two-piece inflatable implants have been removed and replaced by three-piece devices due to patient dissatisfaction. We recommend this two-piece implant in a fairly small percentage of patients.

MULTI-COMPONENT INFLATABLE, THREE-PIECE
Brand Names: *Mentor Alpha I, A.M.S. 700 CX, CXM, ULTREX, Ultrex-plus*

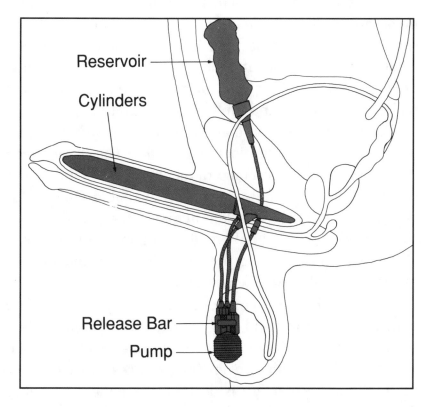

Figure 8 - "Three-Piece Inflatable Prosthesis: Mentor Alpha I"

The introduction of the inflatable prosthesis was made in 1973. Over the last twenty-plus years, inflatable implants have undergone continual improvement. In their beginning stages, the mechanical success rate was 30% in the first five years. This meant that seven of ten implants had to be repaired within 5 years of implantation. Now, some of the devices have a remarkable mechanical reliability rate of 96% in the first five years!

Inflatable penile implants are the most successful imitation of a natural erection that currently exists. It also should be noted that in 1988, the multi-component inflatable passed malleable prostheses in sales for the first time, despite a three-fold price difference, indicating widespread patient and physician acceptance.

There is no question that the "gold standard" of penile implants is the three-piece inflatable. The three-piece inflatables have the best ratio of mechanical reliability and patient satisfaction of any prosthesis available. This multi-component inflatable implant achieves the best erection, a truly rigid, thick, natural erection in almost all men. It is virtually undetectable to the eye when soft and usually cannot be easily noted when feeling the penis.

These devices are composed of two cylinders in the penis, a tiny pump in the scrotum and a fluid filled reservoir located behind the pubic bone. The hydraulic system is filled with two to three ounces (60-100cc) of fluid. When an erection is desired, the patient squeezes the pump implanted in his scrotum, which moves fluid from the reservoir into the penile cylinders. An erection develops which can be maintained as long as desired, even all night! When the patient and his partner have achieved satisfaction, the pump release valve is pressed and the fluid is transferred back into the reservoir. *Patient satisfaction with inflatable implants is the highest of any available treatment for impotence.*

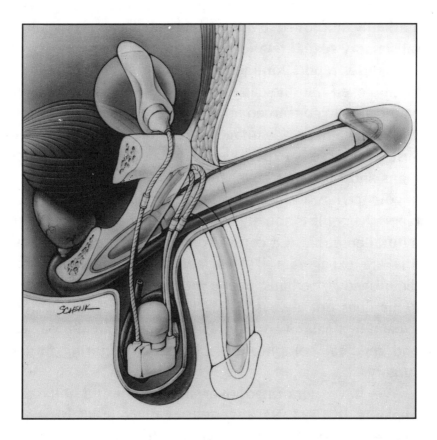

Figure 9 - "Three-Piece Inflatable Prosthesis: A.M.S. 700 CX"

Ninety-five percent of our patients reported "very satisfied" after one year of use as compared to 50% with injection therapy and 33% with vacuum constriction devices. Many patients express to us that they only wished they'd "done it sooner."

We've seen patients turn their lives around after prosthesis implantation. They've stopped smoking, had their teeth fixed, and lost weight. Their quality of life was markedly improved by the ability to have predictable, satisfactory sexual relations with their partners.

Spouses report comments ranging from "no difference" to "improved," to "he can last longer." Only rarely (3%) do partners seem concerned about this "unnatural" assistance.

Despite these advantages, there are some negatives. First, the device is expensive. Fortunately, most insurance plans and Medicare cover the cost of implantation when impotence has a physical cause. Secondly, some patients report the penis is sometimes not as long as their previous natural erection. (Of course some men's memories about this are exaggerated!) This feeling that the length has diminished is, perhaps, due to the fact that the head of the penis does not always inflate with the implant but does expand in a natural erection. Finally, mechanical breakage and medical complication can occur requiring further surgery.

We have performed over three thousand inflatable implants. In 1993, 95% were three-piece inflatables. We utilize most of the devices we have discussed but prefer the *Mentor Alpha I* (Fig. 8) and the *A.M.S.* inflatables for most patients (Fig. 9).

For routine implantation in a patient without previous

penile surgery, there are different reasons, including patient preferences and patient anatomy that help make the decisions about the types of prosthesis implanted. These penile prostheses, being a dynamic, hydraulic system for the most part, can be subject to breakage, and so there is this slight risk in having surgery.

REVISION SURGERY

At the present time, we cannot consider the inflatable prosthesis a lifetime device in most men. At some point in future years, the device may require revision, despite excellent mechanical reliability demonstrated by our recent statistics. Fortunately, this is much less likely than when the prosthesis was first developed. The dependability of the prosthesis has so greatly improved that the manufacturers now offer substantial product warranties. The A.M.S. and Mentor products as of this writing are covered by a lifetime warranty. These warranties do not cover the cost of hospitalization but do cover prosthesis components if replacement is necessary. For revision surgery, Medicare and most commercial insurers reimburse you, just as they do for the initial implant.

A re-operation is (usually) considerably less complicated than the original surgery and usually requires no more than a correction of a minor hydraulic problem. Most patients report such improved quality of life with a prosthesis that the necessity of a revision causes very little consternation. Penile prosthesis infection, while fortunately a rare happening, almost invariably will require further surgery as well.

PROSTHESIS SAFETY

Recently, the FDA began a re-examination of the twenty years of penile prosthesis history in order to determine if there are any hidden health or psychological problems in the patient population of over 200,000 men who have reversed their impotency with a prosthesis. This information is being compiled diligently by the prosthesis manufacturers. As part of this study, we are researching our recently implanted patients. Specifically, authorities are interested in complications similar to those associated with silicone gel breast implants.

While the study is not complete as of this writing, preliminary results have shown *no* problems to be silicone related. Penile implants have medical grade silicone components as do knee cap, hip joint and heart valve replacements and are filled with saline solution not silicone gel. Since their chemical make-up bears no resemblance to the silicone gel filled breast implants, it's no surprise that there have been no reported instances of "silicone disease" or auto immune diseases. We anticipate when the study is completed, penile implants will still be considered the "gold standard" of impotence therapy.

CHOOSING A SURGEON TO PERFORM PROSTHESIS SURGERY

The implantation of the inflatable multi-component device is more complicated than the malleable, positionable, or self-contained devices. This surgery is usually only performed by urologists who specialize in impotence, and is not generally recommended for the urologist who only performs an occasional implant procedure. Implant manufacturers report that 80% of the inflatable prostheses are performed by only 10% of the urologists in America. It is important to realize that while the skillful urologist can perform this surgery with ease, experience with implants is necessary to achieve optimal results.

When performed by our surgeons, the prosthesis is placed through a one-inch incision on the underside or the topside of the penis. This operation usually takes less than one hour. Other surgeons may approach the implantation through other larger incisions. Our extensive implant experience has reduced what some others would consider major surgery, to an outpatient procedure, most of the time.

MAKING THE DECISION TO HAVE SURGERY

The patient should have knowledge of all treatment methods and feel comfortable prior to starting any form of therapy. Penile prosthesis patients should have full knowledge of other acceptable treatment methods and have considered them prior to making a decision to have surgery. Any problems, questions or fears should be resolved before proceeding with surgery or any other treatment. We believe that more time should be spent discussing with the patient treatment alternatives than in repetitive diagnostic testing.

Obviously, there will be unresolved tensions. For example, if the patient has a penile prosthesis, he will go from a non-sexual situation laden with performance anxiety to a state of being able to have an erection all night long. Sometimes this may represent a threat to his sexual partner. Many women initially feel that they are no longer needed to excite or stimulate their man. These same women may wonder if their newly potent mate will want to find another more attractive or younger partner. Fortunately, in a short time, most couples work out these feelings and report intense satisfaction with their sexual relationships. It is not uncommon for the spouse to report that it has. We have a large stack of "thank you" letters to prove it .

Sexual partners should realize that with today's improvements in penile implants, sexual intercourse can be resumed as a very natural process. Penile prosthesis help to maintain a normal function of the body that otherwise would be severely curtailed. Remember that today, impotence is recognized as usually a physical, not mental problem. *Many patients choose an implant to correct physical impotence, just as they would choose a synthetic joint to repair a knee or hip.*

Despite all the successful statistics and educational literature, some people find it is very difficult to make a decision about a penile prosthesis. To these people we strongly suggest they visit with other impotent patients and their partners, who can diminish their fear and explain how this procedure brought sexual happiness back into their lives. In the next chapter, we'll discuss how to contact these caring individuals. I'd like to end this segment with a case study from a couple who were both hesitant.

CASE STUDY

Bill and his wife Ruth first sought help just as Bill was turning 65 and about to retire. He had been experiencing increasing problems with impotence for about 3 years, and now the impotence was complete. Bill and Ruth were looking forward to spending more time together as they traveled the country. But this sexual dysfunction was making the prospect somewhat distressing—for both of them!

A straightforward evaluation; examination, some blood tests, and a snap-gauge test confirmed a physical cause. After reviewing all the treatment options, Bill and Ruth decided upon a three-piece penile prosthesis. I'll never forget the note I received from them, thanking me for basically turning their lives around. They are extremely pleased. It has been several years. I see Bill once a year for a prostate exam, and he is still doing great. They are traveling the country in a large RV and fully enjoying retirement. Their story is so common, and is one of the reasons we enjoy so much working with men, and with couples, to solve these life problems

Chapter 7

Help Is Available

We began telling you this fact on the first page of this book and we are now going to tell you more than we already have about solving this problem. You don't have to suffer from impotence!

SELECTING A UROLOGIST

We mentioned earlier that many urologists do not focus on the evaluation or treatment of impotence, so the reader is advised to research his urologist with care. Fortunately, most major cities have at least one physician who has made impotence a special interest. These physicians may be located by asking your family physician or contacting the following support groups:

Impotence Institute of America
1-(800) 699-1603
8201 Corporate Drive, Ste. 320
Landover, MD 20785-2229

Impotence Foundation
1-(800) 221-5517
P.O. Box 60260
Santa Barbara, CA 93160

These groups have the name, address and telephone number of every urologist in the United States who specializes in impotence. Call either of these numbers for information on the urologist closest to you. Then, visit them and see if you like them. If not, call for another doctor who specializes in your problem. If it's important to you, please don't delay. Do it now!

Impotents Anonymous (IA), founded by Bruce and Eileen Mackenzie, a support group for impotent men and their partners, is an affiliate of the Impotence Institute (II). With more than 100 IA chapters in the U.S. This group was established so that individuals could discuss topics such as coping with impotence and its effect on ones personality. A quarterly newsletter, reports on impotence research and other literature is provided to IA members. You may reach them through the Impotence Institute of America.

Their meetings provide reassurance in a serious setting, support from medical advisors and mental health professionals, and information from urologists who furnish videotapes and lectures at these meetings. At each meeting, several members who have suffered impotence and received treatment are available to share their experiences. There is no question that sharing experiences helps many sufferers to overcome fear and loss of self-worth. Hopefully, those individuals will then seek professional help.

The Impotence Foundation is an organization that offers information, fellowship and self-help. The Impotence Foundation (IF) was established in 1986 to help impotent men and their partners find a workable solution to their problem. IF is a national information service developed to provide educational information on the treatment of impotence. We both were among the founding urologists of the Impotence Foundation.

Local Impotence Foundation meetings are designed to educate people about their options for possible treatments and are not intended to be ongoing counseling groups. Any man who suffers from impotency is welcome at IF support group meetings; spouses and partners are also invited. There are no association fees or dues.

IF uses a variety of resources to provide information to the general public including distribution of literature, by talking to other men who suffer from impotence and listen to how some of them "fixed their problem", and from various experts in the field such as a urologist, an endocrinologist, an internal medicine doctor, psychologist or sex therapist. IF meetings are usually organized by a local urologist, who serves as an IF Chapter Director.

Above all, support groups let people know that it is okay to feel the way they do. Part of the battle for impotence sufferers is depression and a feeling of hopelessness.

Support group sharing and national media attention have helped make millions.

The condition of impotency and its successful treatment has been brought to the attention of the American public through numerous newspapers across the country, NBC's "Today Show," ABC's "20/20," Gary Collins' "Hour Magazine," *Time* magazine, the "Oprah Winfrey Show," the "Sally Jessy Raphael Show," and the "Phil Donahue Show." On each of these programs, impotence sufferers stress the importance of talking about this embarrassing problem with their partner, your doctor, a friend, and/or support group.

TALKING TO OTHER PATIENTS

Many physicians will also have a list of patients and their partners who are willing to discuss their particular therapy and their experience with it. Many will share the effect that the treatment of impotence has had on their relationship with their spouse or partner.

It is often difficult for patients to make the decision to proceed with any of the common treatment methods, even though they know these are safe methods of dealing with a debilitating problem. Most urologists specializing in impotence have patient educational videotapes available. These videos portray patients discussing their life before and after treatment with a vacuum device, injection therapy or penile implant surgery.

It's easy to understand why implant surgery is often the hardest therapy for a couple to select. Most men try to avoid all types of surgery, much less on such a sensitive organ. We see a common pattern. Most men who learn about the availability of implants want to investigate these devices immediately. Then fear sets in. Even after gathering all the information, talking with the urologist and undergoing diagnostic testing, the prospective patient may end up waiting months—or even years—before deciding to have the surgery. Some men, regretfully, never do.

CONCLUSIONS

There is a tremendous amount of worldwide research going on in the field of impotence. As there are new and meaningful developments available, your urologist will likely be aware of them. As future editions of this book appear, we will endeavor to keep you posted with the new developments. However, keep in mind, that although there may be some, as yet discovered, miracle treatment someday, the treatments now available have provided excellent results for hundreds of thousands of men.

Treatment of impotence is a *quality-of-life* issue for many men—and couples. We believe that almost every man suffering can be helped, and it is our *mission*, if we can think of it that way, to let men, and women, understand this problem and its many solutions.

We're here to help if you request it. This is not a condition that *requires* treatment. But, the heartbreaking part of the story is that many men are not even aware that help is available. We've been able to help almost everyone in our many years in this field. Almost always, there is some type of solution.

We're both hoping that this book both enlightens you on the methods in curing impotency and helps you make a decision to do something about it! Just know that if you want help in recovering from impotence, we, and many other urologic specialists are ready to provide that help.

CASE STUDIES

The following case studies were selected from our files to illustrate common situations experienced by our impotence patients. Names, ages and occupations were changed so that no actual patients are referenced. The reader may find one of these clinical situation *very* familiar.

CASE STUDY #101

Al, a widower in his late seventies, was inactive sexually in the last years of a long marriage. His wife had been stricken with cancer and a warm, loving relationship without sex had sustained them throughout her illness. After she died, Al began to date and noted, to his distress, that his mind was willing but his erection failed him. Eventually, he became involved with a very understanding lady, Denise, who suggested he attend an Impotence Support Group Meeting. There, Al found he was not alone. There were many other individuals his age who had developed and successfully treated this embarrassing problem.

He was referred to a urologist specializing in impotence. After a thorough history and physical, his urologist performed an NPT test which showed no "sleep erections" and pinpointed the diagnosis of physical impotence caused by vascular insufficiency. He underwent penile prosthesis implantation and within three months he and Denise were honeymooning.

This is one of the most common examples of patients in an impotence clinic. The male has ceased sexual activity during the concluding years of a marriage due to illness of his sexual partner. After the loss of the loved one and a suitable period of grieving, the man becomes interested in establishing new relationships. Unfortunately, and often to his great surprise, he has interest in his new lady friend but can't fulfill his desires, or hers, due to impotency. These individuals can profit immensely from impotency therapy, if only they know it is available! The pity is that too many men suffer in silence and their prospective partners are deprived of a healthy, happy new relationship.

CASE STUDY #35

Robert was a 46 year-old businessman whose sexual relationship with his wife had been deteriorating over the past eight years due to his periodic bouts of impotence. Although other aspects of his marriage had seemingly gone untouched through this period, they were now obviously suffering the negative effects of his erectile failure and performance anxiety.

When things became almost hopeless, Robert consulted his urologist who suggested some books on male physiology and sexual functioning. Soon, Robert was learning how to control his feelings of "fear of failure" through relaxation methods. He and his wife began to meet with a marriage counselor who suggested that they communicate more intimately and take more chances in their sexual lives.

They also began attending sexual therapy, where they learned through books and private discussion to explore each other in a calm and pleasurable way. Robert kept track of his progress and began to see a definite improvement. His self-esteem and confidence level increased and his marriage reached a higher level of commitment and sharing. In a short time, Robert was able to improve his long-standing impotency problem.

Sexual counseling is especially effective when couples have a loving relationship and are able to participate in the counseling without assigning blame. Sexual counseling is doomed to failure if the couple's sexual problems are but one expression of a larger picture of incompatibility.

CASE STUDY #81

Charles, a thirty-seven year-old investment banker, was recently divorced and seeking female companionship. He had been desperately lonely for some time until he met Stephanie, an attractive woman in her late thirties. Thrilled with the prospect of a relationship, Charles was blind to Stephanie's shortcomings. They soon began a sexual relationship. Their lovemaking was usually preceded by a night of sustained drinking.

Initially, the relationship was exciting. Then, Charles consistently overindulged in drinking and was eventually unable to perform in bed. Stephanie began to question his performance, even tease him. Fortunately, he associated his feelings of guilt and lack of control with his relationship with Stephanie and started to date other women. He entered into a more stable relationship with another lady, significantly decreased his alcohol consumption and resumed a normal sex life.

Alcohol consumption is one of the leading causes of temporary impotence. It is important to note that the likelihood of impotence associated with alcohol consumption increases with age. Some men as they become older develop very high sensitivity to alcohol so that even one or two drinks will depress the ability to perform sexually. The temporary impotence is usually reversed if sexual intercourse is performed without "having a few drinks."

CASE STUDY #91

Hank, a college professor, attended a free screening during *Prostate Cancer Awareness Week*. A digital rectal exam and a blood test called PSA were performed. Hank was called back a week later and a prostate ultrasound and biopsy were performed. He was found to have localized cancer of the prostate. Luckily the cancer had not spread yet and was found very early due to the screening clinic.

Hank underwent the surgical removal of his cancerous gland by an operation called *radical prostatectomy*. His urologist told him he had a 60% chance of being left impotent after the operation.

Six months after the operation, Hank was thought to be cured of cancer and back to a full and productive life-style. Unfortunately, his erections were very poor. He and his wife had tried valiantly to stimulate an erection. Hank's penis would only get "fat" but never rigid enough to penetrate. Hank's urologist prescribed a vacuum device to see if this would help the couple. The vacuum device improved rigidity enough for penetration but orgasm was difficult and the erection was not natural to Hank. He also disliked interrupting foreplay to activate the device.

Next, his urologist prescribed a program of "injection erection." This was initially successful, producing natural erections, but then Hank got an erection which persisted for six hours. This also necessitated an extremely embarrassing trip to the Emergency Room to get therapy to reverse the erection (priapism).

Hank's urologist then referred him to one of the authors to consider inflatable implant surgery. Since Hank had tried and failed with other common treatments, no further diagnostic tests were necessary and the implantation was performed soon after the first visit. The surgery was done as an outpatient procedure with minimal discomfort, and within a few short weeks Hank and his wife were once again enjoying an active sex life.

While the operation for cancer of the prostate has been designed to spare the nerves controlling erection, impotence is still a common complication of radical prostatectomy. It is common for vacuum device and injection erection to be prescribed early in the post-operative period. Eventually, however, the usual therapy to provide a permanent solution to the problem is a penile prosthesis. This case also illustrates a common practice among urologists, that of referring their patients interested in an implant to one of their colleagues who has greater experi-

ence with this surgical procedure.

CASE STUDY #15

Steven, a seventy year-old retiree, had been impotent for several years before suffering a severe heart attack and being diagnosed with arteriosclerosis. He had been suffering heart problems for many years prior to his heart attack but never knew his impotency was merely another symptom of generalized hardening of all the arteries in his body.

After a serious hospitalization, his cardiologist ruled out coronary bypass surgery due to other health conditions. He was treated with medication and soon felt stronger than anytime in recent years. He felt so good he began to think about resuming sexual activity. He and his wife had shared an intimate sexual relationship prior to his impotency and heart problems, and were overjoyed to discover that impotency could be reversed.

His cardiac condition meant increased surgical risk for penile implantation, and because he was on blood thinner medication, injection therapy was not possible. Therefore, his cardiologist and urologist recommended a therapy which was non-invasive.

Steven obtained a vacuum device from his urologist and planned to use it until his physicians cleared him for implant surgery. To his surprise, he and his wife enjoyed sexual intercourse so much they continued with the vacuum device even after his cardiologist said he was an acceptable surgical risk.

Vacuum constriction devices are particularly useful when the couple is highly motivated and injection therapy or penile implantation is not advisable. In our experience, the idea of using these devices is often more distasteful than the actual use. If a couple is forced to use these devices because better therapies are not available, the anxiety may vanish and satisfying pleasure can be derived.

CASE STUDY #69

Rodney, a young bull rider in his mid-twenties, suffered a serious injury while practicing for a state-wide rodeo. Doctors soon discovered that Rodney had severely damaged his spinal cord, leaving him partially paralyzed and almost totally impotent. Emotionally devastated, Rodney was unable to maintain an erection throughout sexual intercourse. In fact, it was becoming more and more difficult for Rodney to achieve an erection at all.

Since he had only recently married, Rodney's desire to rebuild his sex life was as important to him as therapy to regain other physical functions. When his urologist told him that implantation of a penile prosthesis was an option, Rodney had doubts. He began a program of injection erections immediately which kept his spirits high during his difficult physical rehabilitation. His wife remained very supportive throughout the ordeal. Once fully rehabilitated, Rodney opted for inflatable prosthesis implantation. Today, Rodney and his wife report much happiness with their quality of life.

Neurogenic impotence, such as in spinal cord injury, is

generally treated quite successfully by the choice of injection therapy. Because the injected medication dosages are so small, the chance of complication is small. This patient might have continued on injection therapy indefinitely if he had not wished to undergo penile prosthesis implantation.

CASE STUDY #92

A heavy smoker, Fred noted he had difficulty keeping his erection after he reached fifty. Eventually he began to fail so often he started to avoid sexual situations. When forced by his wife to attempt sexual intercourse, he was totally unable to get an erection. With his marriage of 35 years in severe jeopardy, Fred sought help. His urologist found Fred had mild vascular impotence compounded severely by performance anxiety.

Stopping smoking and reassurance helped Fred initially, but then he failed again. Eventually, an "injection erection" program was started and Fred and his wife reported great satisfaction with this therapy. The injections were needed only occasionally. Knowing he could use them if necessary virtually eliminated his performance anxiety. Fred understands that eventually his vascular impotence will cause complete erectile failure. But, for now, a loving relationship and the backup availability of injection medication have greatly improved his sex life.

Fred illustrates an important use of "injection erection" therapy as a stand-by treatment in men who are partially functional. Although the ability to achieve erection is impaired, these men may perform for years without steady therapy, provided the performance anxiety can be relieved. Vacuum devices can also be useful in these cases.

CLOSING COMMENTS

We hope our efforts in writing this book were helpful to you. In reading over parts of it, it may seem that some of our treatments are painful and that they are not guaranteed to work. The fact of the matter is that *almost all* the treatments are not painful and a vast percentage of them do work!

For insurance reasons, we say "almost" and "most of the time" because there will always be one person, usually an opportunist, who will sue us for trying to help them overcome a debilitating problem. We are only human, and we can never completely predict how every man will respond to any given treatment, or precisely how one may recover from surgery.

Also, we are not salesmen, but medical doctors; urologists who specialize in impotency. And although our practices are full, we will always find time to consult and direct you because we care. We truly do.

Good luck, and God bless,

David F. Mobley   Steven K. Wilson
Houston, Texas   Van Buren, Arkansas

To make an appointment with Dr. David Mobley:
920 Frostwood, Suite 610
Houston, Texas 77024-2414
(713) 932-1819

For Dr. Steven Wilson:
2010 Chestnut
Van Buren, Arkansas 72956
(501) 474-1225

Other Books by Swan Publishing

HOW NOT TO BE LONELY . . . If you're about to marry, recently divorced or widowed, want to forgive, forget or both, this is an excellent book to read. Candid, positive, entertaining and informative (over 2 million copies sold) . . . . $ 9.95

HOW NOT TO BE LONELY *TONIGHT* . . . aimed at the *MALE* reader. Other than being courageous and strong, smart women want their man to be sensitive, caring, and understanding. "The" book to give to your man. Or, for men who really want to learn what turns the modern woman on . . . . $ 9.95

NEW FATHER'S BABY GUIDE . . . The "perfect" gift for ALL new fathers. Tells (dummy dad) about Lamaze classes, burping, feeding and changing the baby plus 40 side-splitting drawings. Most of all, it tells dad how to SPOIL mom! . . . . $ 9.95

YOUR FRONT YARD . . . information about plants, trees, grass, shrubs, pesticides, fertilizers; everything you need to know about what to plant and how to take care of it in southern climates, written by gardening expert, John Burrow. . . . . $ 9.95

HOME IMPROVEMENT (Homeowner's Most Often Asked Questions) written by home improvement celebrity talk show and television host, Tom Tynan, with candor and humor and stacked with information about lighting, roofing, electrical, painting, air conditioning and hundreds of answers to questions that will help you fix things around the house . . . .$ 9.95

BUILDING & REMODELING, also by Tom Tynan on whether you should (or shouldn't) build and/or remodel on your own., Choosing a contractor, subs, permits, loans, etc ...... $ 9.95

BUYING & SELLING A HOME, Volume 3 by Tom Tynan tells you secrets to do it all. Realtors buy this book and it will help anyone who is buying or getting a home ready to sell ... $ 9.95

VEGETABLE GARDENING *SPRING & FALL*, by John Burrow, tells about growing vegetables if you live in the city, the country, an apartment or town home. And, how to do it easily and successfully and have fun while doing it .... $ 9.95

KEEP IT UP (Due in September of 1995, written by Dr. David F. Mobley) tells how To PREVENT Impotence! The book goes into detail on how to avoid and/or delay impotence. Everything in the book is positive, even the title! A terrific book for men and women .... $ 9.95

Each book is $9.95 per copy, plus $2.90 for shipping and handling costs, (or $12.85 per book).

Dr. David F. Mobley is available for personal appearances, luncheons, banquets, seminars, etc. He is entertaining and informative. Call (713) 388-2547 for cost and availability.

Dr. Mobley's show airs over KSEV, 700 AM on your radio dial in Houston, each Monday thru Friday from 1-2pm.

For a copy of *Reversing Impotence Forever,* send a personal check or money order for $12.85 ($9.95 plus $2.90 shipping and handling) per copy to: Swan Publishing, 126 Live Oak, Alvin, TX, 77511. Allow 7-10 days for delivery; 3-5 days for delivery in Texas.

To order by major credit card 24 hours a day call: **(713) 268-6776** or long distance **1-800-966-8962**

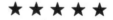

Libraries—Bookstores—Quantity Orders

Swan Publishing, 126 Live Oak, Alvin, TX 77511
Call (713) 388-2547 or FAX (713) 585-3738